Eat Healthy, Burn Good, Live Better! [3 in 1]

Eat Dozens of Delicious Mediterranean Recipes, Customize Your Workouts and Regain Your Lost Shape!

Anphora Cooper

Text Copyright © Anphora Cooper

Legal & Disclaimer

Upon using the contents and information contained in this book, you agree to hold harmless the Author from and against any damages, costs, and expenses, including any legal fees potentially resulting from the application of any of the information provided by this book. This disclaimer applies to any loss, damages or injury caused by the use and application, whether directly or indirectly, of any advice or information presented, whether for breach of contract, tort, negligence, personal injury, criminal intent, or under any other cause of action.

You agree to accept all risks of using the information presented inside this book.

You agree that by continuing to read this book, where appropriate and/or necessary, you shall consult a professional (including but not limited to your doctor, attorney, or financial advisor or such other advisor as needed) before using any of the suggested remedies, techniques, or information in this book.

Contents

The Mediterranean Diet Cookbook with Pictures

The 15-Day Men's Health Book of 15-Minute Workouts

The 15-Day Women's Health Book of 15-Minute Workouts

The Mediterranean Diet Cookbook with Pictures

Tens of Tasty Recipes to Shed Weight and Feel Great in 2021

Anphora Cooper

Contents

Introduction

Many people may think about "a diet" as a particular weight reduction plan; however diet just alludes to the sorts and measures of food an individual eats. An empowering diet should incorporate equilibrium of a few nutrition classes, as no single gathering can give all the body requires to great wellbeing. Settling on healthy food decisions decreases an individual's danger of numerous persistent medical issues, including cardiovascular illness, two types of diabetes, and disease. There is an abundance of data accessible, so planning a reasonable, restorative diet can feel overpowering. All things considered, a couple of straightforward changes can make a diet more nutritious and decrease the danger of numerous clinical issues. Eating great is central to acceptable wellbeing and prosperity. Healthy eating causes us to keep a healthy weight and lessens our danger of type 2 diabetes, hypertension, elevated cholesterol and the danger of creating cardiovascular sickness and a few tumors.

Healthy diet

Healthy eating has numerous different advantages. At the point when we eat well we rest better, have more energy and better fixation and this all amounts to better, more joyful lives! Healthy eating ought to be a pleasant social encounter. At the point when kids and youngsters eat and drink well they get all the fundamental supplements they require for legitimate development and improvement, and build up a decent connection with food and other social abilities.

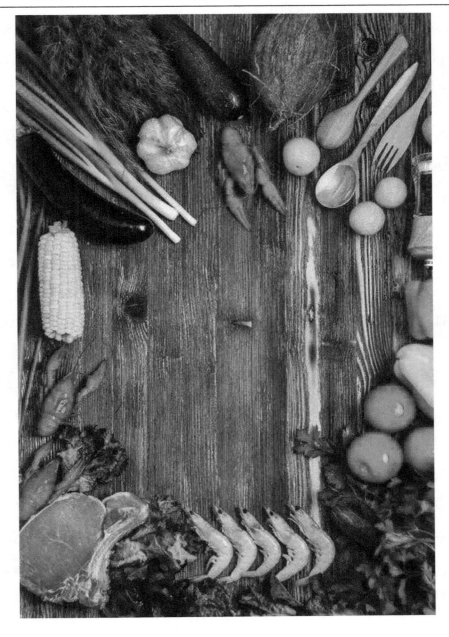

Healthy diet isn't tied in with removing nourishments it's tied in with eating a wide assortment of food sources in the perfect adds up to give your body what it needs. There are no single nourishments you should eat or menus you need to follow to eat strongly. You simply need to ensure you get the correct equilibrium of various food sources. Healthy eating for youngsters and youngsters ought to consistently incorporate a scope of fascinating and scrumptious food that can make up a healthy, differed and adjusted diet, as opposed to denying them certain nourishments and beverages. Albeit everything food sources can be remembered for a healthy diet, this won't be valid for individuals on uncommon/clinical diets.

Healthy diets assists individuals with keeping up and improve their overall wellbeing. It is imperative to allow the correct supplements every day to acquire a healthy diet. Supplements can be gotten in numerous food sources and a huge number of diet plans. It is significant that individuals watch their admission of diet plans. It is significant that individuals watch their admission of food to keep a healthy diet. Having an unhealthy diet can be a significant danger factor for various persistent infections including hypertension, weight, and diabetes. It's vital to realize how to bring down hypertension since it's a condition that builds the danger for coronary episode, stroke, kidney disappointment, and other medical issues. The decisions we make in our way of life can go far towards forestalling hypertension. Individuals, who don't as of now have hypertension, should get comfortable with healthy propensities to diminish their danger of truly getting it. Individuals, who as of now have hypertension, ought to quickly begin healthy propensities to bring down their pulse and decline their danger of creating significant complexities. Overseeing pressure is significant in light of the fact that pressure can cause significant damage anybody and it can assume a critical part in hypertension.

Importance of healthy diet

The significance of devouring the appropriate diet can't be focused on enough, particularly as we age. The nourishments that we decide to eat every day can have various impacts on the brain and body and can have a tremendous effect on our mind-set and ways of life. Albeit as a rule we may end up battling to oppose that thicker style skillet select pizza, picking a better option can truly pay off! Rehearsing a healthy diet and reliably devouring the correct supplements can have five significant effects, among numerous others!

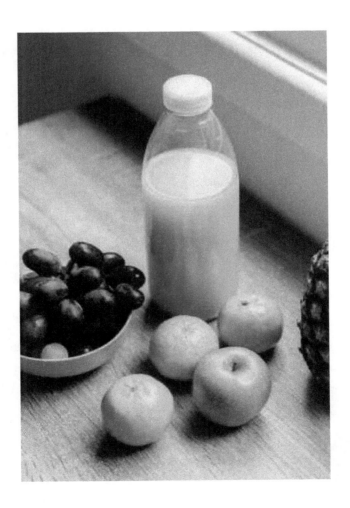

Keep up Normal Body Function

As we age, you may see that you can't hear very too or experience difficulty recollecting straightforward notes that in earlier years would have been no issue! In all honesty, our diet can significantly affect numerous substantial capacities. These including your five detect, pH level, pulse, glucose level, the capacity to modify tissues and your equilibrium. Rehearsing a healthy diet can assist you with keeping up these body capacities as you keep on maturing.

Keep up Healthy Weight

This one ought to be an easy decision. In the event that you eat seared food consistently you won't seem as though the conditioned bodies you find in wellness magazines. Not exclusively does eating healthy hold your weight down, it additionally lessens the danger of coronary illness, diabetes and irregular circulatory strain.

Forestall Diseases

At the point when you eat a balanced diet including an assortment of foods grown from the ground, lean proteins and entire grains that are low in trans and soaked fat, you are diminishing the danger of becoming ill and creating persistent infections like cardiovascular and diabetes.

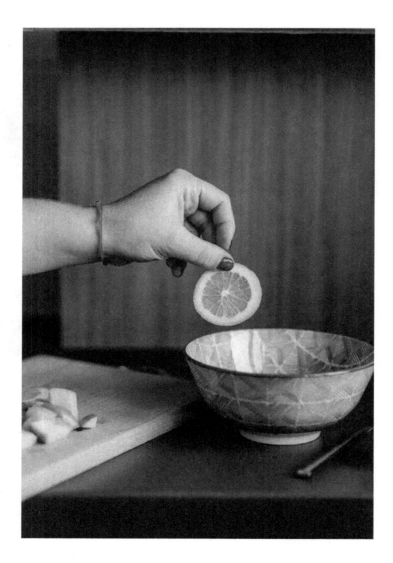

Mind-set and Energy

An even diet influences your body and its capacities, however your psyche also. Nutrients assume a part in the activity of synapses and insufficiencies that can prompt gloom and state of mind problems. Great nourishment can likewise support your energy level, which than thusly can help you complete your day by day schedule easily, eventually bringing about a superior mind-set – so eat great food!

Give Stress Relief

Like the effect nutrients have on your state of mind, legitimate sustenance can likewise give pressure alleviation by lessening the results of medicine, boosting the insusceptible framework, and can assist you with keeping up quieting and adapting capacities.

WHAT and WHEN to Eat

With presence of mind the vast majority can sort out what to eat and what not to eat. Leafy foods give the fundamental nutrients expected to a healthy diet and are in every case bravo. Lean proteins, for example, egg whites, yogurt, salmon, fish and other ocean nourishments and chicken bosom are generally incredible models. Leafy foods, sugars, lean protein, and nutrients and minerals are for the most part key fixings to a healthy way of life. Shockingly, WHAT you eat is a large portion of the fight. The WHEN is nearly pretty much as significant as the substance of the food sources you pick. It is significant not to over-eat, implying that you should customer more modest bits of food for the duration of the day. Breakfast, lunch and supper ought not to be skipped, yet make certain to nibble on a yogurt, banana or fiber bar in the middle of dinners. Eating more modest parts of food all through the whole day will accelerate your digestion and keep you strong and smart.

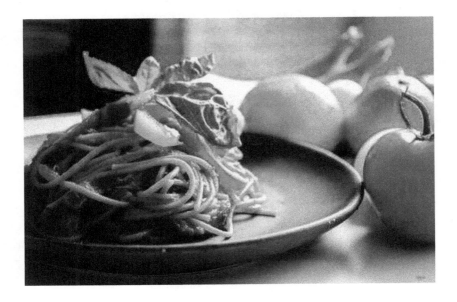

Balanced Diet

An individual needs proper measures of proteins, minerals, and supplements in a balanced diet. It is very essential for the smooth working of our body. In the event that we devour a balanced diet consistently, we will consistently stay healthy. It reduces any odds of becoming sick. Additionally, a balanced diet likewise supports our insusceptibility framework.

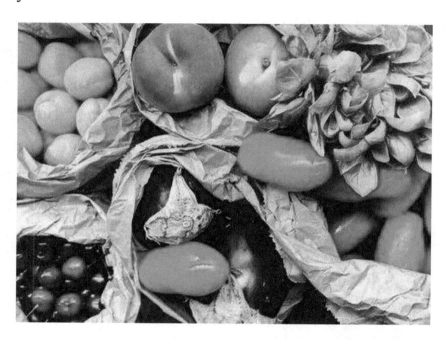

Significance of a Balanced Diet

The vast majority accept that a balanced diet is certainly the way in to a healthy way of life. It is appropriately accepted as even researchers say as much. At the point when we generally devour a balanced diet, we will keep up our physical just as emotional well-being. A balanced diet should contain the legitimate food sources that are burned-through in well-suited amounts. An ideal balanced diet is made out of carbs, proteins, fats, minerals, high fiber substance, nutrients, and then some.

In addition, these days the pattern of shoddy nourishment is staying put. Individuals are not taking a balanced diet rather eating a wide range of unsafe nourishments. It is a higher priority than at any other time to enlighten individuals regarding the significance of a balanced diet. You can't simply practice and anticipate that your body should remain fit. A balanced diet is significant for that.

Above all, it is known as a 'balanced' diet since it requires all the food sources to be eaten in a balanced way. For example, in the event that you admission a lot of sugars and a little measure of protein, at that point that won't be known as a balanced diet, regardless of whether you are eating the correct nourishments. The equilibrium should be kept up for that.

Besides, these days the pattern of lousy nourishment is setting down deep roots. Individuals are not taking a balanced diet rather eating a wide range of hurtful food sources. It is a higher priority than at any other time to inform individuals regarding the significance of a balanced diet. You can't simply practice and anticipate that your body should remain fit. A balanced diet is vital for that.

In particular, it is known as a 'balanced' diet since it requires all the food sources to be eaten in a balanced way. For example, in the event that you intake a lot of sugars and a little measure of protein, at that point that won't be known as a balanced diet, regardless of whether you are eating the correct food sources. The equilibrium should be kept up for that.

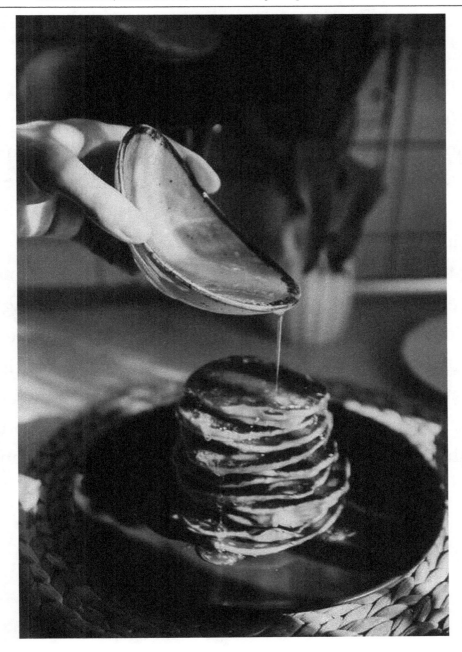

The Mediterranean Diet

In the event that you've at any point conversed with someone after they've ventured out to a country like Italy or Greece, they presumably referenced how delightful the food was. Food is one of the more normal affiliations with nations that encompass the Mediterranean Sea; and naturally so. The food this locale produces is striking to such an extent that there is a diet based off it, companied with perpetual examination expounding the medical advantages it obliges. Fittingly named The Mediterranean Diet, this gathering of food sources including fish, natural products, vegetables, beans, high fiber breads, entire grains, nuts, olive oil and red wine are focused to help forestall various infections just as advance wellbeing in various areas of the body. This book will address every segment, advantage, and precautionary measure of the Mediterranean diet, top to bottom, all with a primary spotlight on the dietary variables.

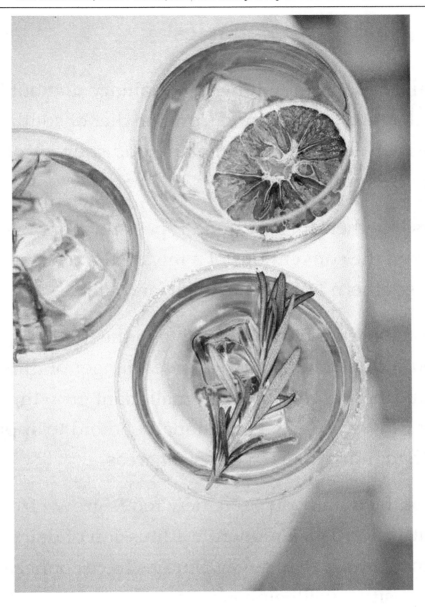

Basics

The Mediterranean diet is anything but a solitary diet but instead an eating design that takes motivation from the diet of southern European nations. There is an accentuation on plant food sources, olive oil, fish, poultry, beans, and grains.

The diet draws together the basic food types and empowering propensities from the conventions of a few distinct locales, including Greece, Spain, southern France, Portugal, and Italy.

Studies propose that individuals who live in the Mediterranean zone or follow the Mediterranean diet have a lower danger of different infections, including weight, diabetes, malignant growth, and cardiovascular illness. They are additionally bound to appreciate a more extended life than individuals in different areas.

Key elements of the diet incorporate new foods grown from the ground, unsaturated fats, slick fish, a moderate admission of dairy, and a low utilization of meat and added sugar. Studies have connected these elements with positive wellbeing results.

Mediterranean Diet
sweets, red meat
monthly or small amounts
dairy, eggs, poultry
daily to weekly
fish, seafood
a few times per week
olive oil
daily servings
vegetables, fruit
daily servings
cereals, beans, legumes, nuts, seeds
daily servings

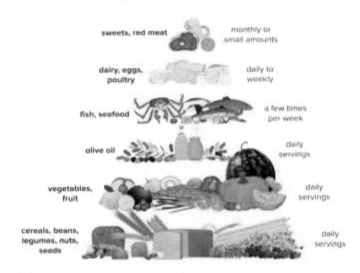

Facts about the Mediterranean Diet

A diet routine that is acquiring in prevalence in numerous pieces of the world depends on the feasting practices of individuals that populate the Mediterranean district. Numerous individuals have known about the Mediterranean diet however are not especially acquainted with a portion of the particulars of the eating schedule.

To help you in getting more acquainted with the Mediterranean diet, a thought of eight valuable realities in regards to the components of this eating routine can be generally useful to you. Obviously, these are just some fundamental arguments about this important dieting schedule. Before you set out on such a diet plan, including the Mediterranean diet, you need to set aside the effort to talk with your doctor to verify that a proposed routine is suitable to your clinical status.

Eight interesting Facts about the Mediterranean Diet

The vital components of the Mediterranean diet are new products of the soil, entire grains, olive oil, fish, and wine with some restraint. As a result of this mix, the Mediterranean diet is one of the best dieting regimens to be discovered anyplace on the planet.

Meat and creature items are burned-through in limited quantities in the Mediterranean diet. Undoubtedly, when meat is incorporated inside the diet conspire; it is poultry or fish in by far most of cases.

Red meat is definitely not a staple in the Mediterranean diet and is seldom eaten by disciples to this dieting schedule. Individuals who really populate the nations around the Mediterranean Sea are once in a while seen eating red meats of any sort. Likewise, dairy items are utilized just sparingly inside the Mediterranean diet. For instance, if milk is remembered for a dinner or in the arrangement of food, it is of the low fat or non-fat assortment. Eggs are once in a while remembered for Mediterranean dinners. Without a doubt, a substantial egg -eater is one who has four eggs per week.

With the moderate utilization of fish, the Mediterranean diet permits followers an enormous wellspring of Omega-3 unsaturated fats. Examination has shown that a diet flush with Omega-3 unsaturated fats attempts to forestall coronary illness, stroke and even a few tumors.

Numerous ignorant individuals can be discovered offering the expression: "The Mediterranean diet simply isn't for me - it is excessively high in fat." In truth, the Mediterranean diet is high in particular sorts of fat. Upwards to 35 to a little less than half of the calories taken in through this diet do come from fat. Notwithstanding, the Mediterranean diet is strikingly low in immersed fat. It is immersed fat that has contrary results on an individual's wellbeing and prosperity.

The diet depends intensely on olive oil. (This is the essential motivation behind why the diet is higher in fat than one may expect.) Olive oil is demonstrated to build the degree of HDL cholesterol (otherwise called "great cholesterol").

The Mediterranean diet is incredibly high in cell reinforcements and fiber, two components that have been demonstrated to be useful in forestalling coronary illness and a few kinds of malignancy.

The dietary acts of the Mediterranean locale follow their birthplaces back to the times of the Roman Republic and the Roman Empire, starting in about the Fourth Century BC.

The Mediterranean diet was the fate of more global interest in present day times as right on time as 1945. A clinical specialist named Ancel Keys was answerable for empowering his own patients in the United States to go to the Mediterranean diet conspires. His support expanded the consciousness of the Mediterranean diet in different nations around the planet also.

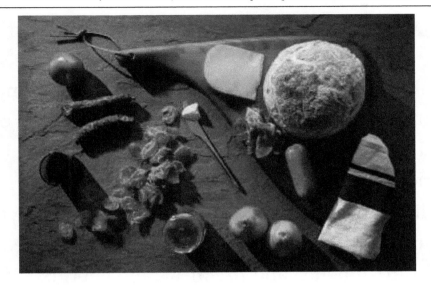

Health Benefits of a Mediterranean diet

- A customary Mediterranean diet comprising of enormous amounts of new foods grown from the ground, nuts, fish, and olive oil—combined with active work—can lessen your danger of genuine mental and actual medical conditions by:

- **Forestalling coronary illness and strokes**. Following a Mediterranean diet restricts your admission of refined breads, handled nourishments, and red meat, and energizes drinking red wine rather than hard alcohol—all factors that can help forestall coronary illness and stroke.

- **Keeping you spry**. In case you're a more seasoned grown-up, the supplements acquired with a Mediterranean diet may diminish your danger of creating muscle shortcoming and different indications of delicacy by around 70%.

- **Lessening the danger of Alzheimer's**. Exploration proposes that the Mediterranean diet may improve cholesterol, glucose levels, and generally vein wellbeing, which thus may diminish your danger of Alzheimer's sickness or dementia.

- **Dividing the danger of Parkinson's infection.** The undeniable degrees of cell reinforcements in the Mediterranean diet can keep cells from going through a harming interaction called oxidative pressure, subsequently cutting the danger of Parkinson's infection fifty-fifty.

- **Expanding life span.** By lessening your danger of creating coronary illness or malignant growth with the Mediterranean diet, you're diminishing your danger of death at whatever stage in life by 20%.

- **Ensuring against type 2- diabetes**. A Mediterranean diet is wealthy in fiber which processes gradually, forestalls gigantic swings in glucose, and can assist you with keeping a healthy weight.

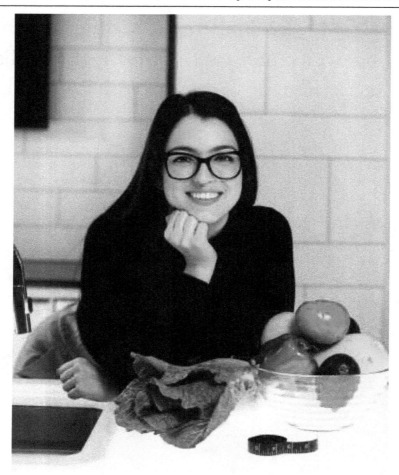

Tips:

- **Eat:** vegetables, organic products, nuts, seeds, vegetables, potatoes, entire grains, breads, spices, flavors, fish, fish and additional virgin olive oil.
- **Eat with some restraint**: Poultry, eggs, cheddar and yogurt.
- **Eat just infrequently**: Red meat.

Try not to eat: Sugar-improved refreshments, added sugars, prepared meat, refined grains, refined oils and other exceptionally handled nourishments.

Dodge These Unhealthy Foods

You ought to keep away from these unhealthy food sources and fixings:

- **Added sugar**: Soda, confections, frozen yogurt, table sugar and numerous others.
- **Refined grains**: White bread, pasta made with refined wheat, and so on
- **Tran's fats**: Found in margarine and different prepared food sources.
- **Refined oils**: Soybean oil, canola oil, cottonseed oil and others.

Prepared meat: Processed wieners, franks, and so forth

Exceptionally prepared food sources: Anything named "low-fat" or "diet" or which seems as though it was made in a manufacturing plant.

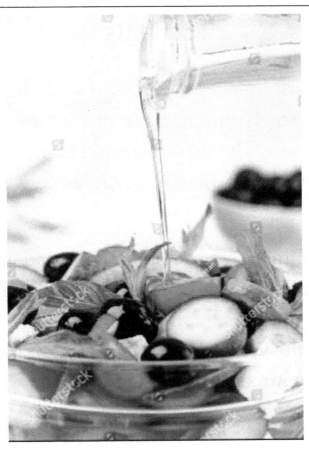

Nourishments to Eat

Precisely which nourishments have a place with the Mediterranean diet is disputable, incompletely on the grounds that there is such variety between various nations. The diet inspected by most examinations is high in healthy plant food sources and moderately low in creature nourishments.

Notwithstanding, eating fish and fish is suggested at any rate double seven days. The Mediterranean way of life likewise includes customary active work, offering dinners to others and getting a charge out of life. You should put together your diet with respect to these healthy, natural Mediterranean food sources:

- **Vegetables**: Tomatoes, broccoli, kale, spinach, onions, cauliflower, carrots, Brussels sprouts, cucumbers, and so on
- **Organic products**: Apples, bananas, oranges, pears, strawberries, grapes, dates, figs, melons, peaches, and so forth
- **Nuts and seeds**: Almonds, pecans, macadamia nuts, hazelnuts, cashews, sunflower seeds, pumpkin seeds, and so forth
- **Vegetables:** Beans, peas, lentils, beats, peanuts, chickpeas, and so forth.
- Tubers: Potatoes, yams, turnips, sweet potatoes, and so forth
- **Entire grains:** Whole oats, earthy colored rice, rye, grain, corn, buckwheat, entire wheat, entire grain bread and pasta.
- **Fish and fish:** Salmon, sardines, trout, fish, mackerel, shrimp, shellfish, mollusks, crab, mussels, and so forth
- **Poultry:** Chicken, duck, turkey, and so forth
- **Eggs:** Chicken, quail and duck eggs.

- **Dairy:** Cheese, yogurt, Greek yogurt, and so forth
- **Spices and flavors**: Garlic, basil, mint, rosemary, sage, nutmeg, cinnamon, pepper, and so forth

Healthy Fats: Extra virgin olive oil, olives, avocados and avocado oil.

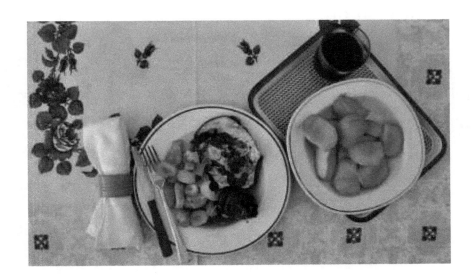

What to Drink

Water ought to be your go-to drink on a Mediterranean diet. This diet additionally incorporates moderate measures of red wine around 1 glass each day. Nonetheless, this is totally discretionary, and wine ought to be dodged by anybody with liquor addiction or issues controlling their utilization.

Espresso and tea are additionally totally worthy, yet you ought to dodge sugar-improved drinks and organic product juices, which are high in sugar.

A Mediterranean Sample Menu for 1 Week

The following is an example menu for multi week on the Mediterranean diet. Don't hesitate to change the bits and food decisions dependent on your own necessities and inclinations.

Monday

- **Breakfast**: Greek yogurt with strawberries and oats.
- **Lunch**: Whole-grain sandwich with vegetables.
- **Supper**: A fish serving of mixed greens, wearing olive oil. A piece of organic product for dessert.

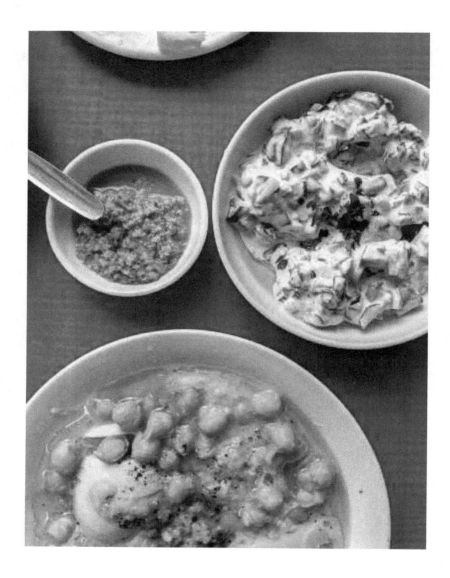

Tuesday

- **Breakfast:** Oatmeal with raisins.
- **Lunch**: Leftover fish serving of mixed greens from the prior night.

Supper: Salad with tomatoes, olives and feta cheddar.

Wednesday

- **Breakfast**: Omelet with veggies, tomatoes and onions. A piece of organic product.
- **Lunch:** Whole-grain sandwich, with cheddar and new vegetables.

Supper: Mediterranean lasagna.

Thursday

- **Breakfast:** Yogurt with cut leafy foods.
- **Lunch:** Leftover lasagna from the prior night.

Supper: Broiled salmon, presented with earthy colored rice and vegetables.

Friday

- **Breakfast**: Eggs and vegetables, seared in olive oil.
- **Lunch:** Greek yogurt with strawberries, oats and nuts.

Supper: Grilled sheep, with serving of mixed greens and heated potato.

Saturday

- **Breakfast**: Oatmeal with raisins, nuts and an apple.
- **Lunch:** Whole-grain sandwich with vegetables.

Supper: Mediterranean pizza made with entire wheat, finished off with cheddar, vegetables and olives.

Sunday

- **Breakfast:** Omelet with veggies and olives.
- **Lunch:** Leftover pizza from the prior night.
- **Supper**: Grilled chicken, with vegetables and a potato. Natural product for dessert.

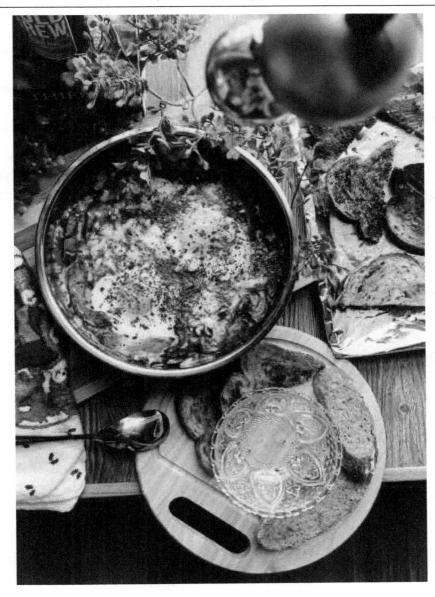

Healthy Mediterranean Snacks

You don't have to eat multiple dinners each day. In any case, on the off chance that you become hungry between dinners, there are a lot of healthy nibble choices:

- A modest bunch of nuts.
- A piece of organic product.
- Carrots or child carrots.
- A few berries or grapes.
- Extras from the prior night.
- Greek yogurt.

Apple cuts with almond margarine.

A Simple Shopping List for the Diet

It is consistently a smart thought to shop at the border of the store. That is typically where the entire food sources are. Continuously attempt to pick the most un-handled alternative. Natural is ideal, however just on the off chance that you can undoubtedly bear the cost of it.

- **Vegetables**: Carrots, onions, broccoli, spinach, kale, garlic, and so on
- **Natural products:** Apples, bananas, oranges, grapes, and so forth
- **Berries:** Strawberries, blueberries, and so on
- **Frozen veggies:** Choose blends in with healthy vegetables.
- **Grains:** Whole-grain bread, entire grain pasta, and so on
- **Vegetables:** Lentils, beats, beans, and so on
- **Nuts:** Almonds, pecans, cashews, and so on
- **Seeds**: Sunflower seeds, pumpkin seeds, and so forth
- **Sauces**: Sea salt, pepper, turmeric, cinnamon, and so forth
- **Fish**: Salmon, sardines, mackerel, trout.
- Shrimp and shellfish.
- Potatoes and yams.
- Cheddar.
- Greek yogurt.
- Chicken.
- Fed or omega-3 enhanced eggs.
- Olives.

Extra virgin olive oil.

It's ideal to clear all unhealthy enticements from your home, including soft drinks, frozen yogurt, candy, baked goods, white bread, saltines and prepared food sources.

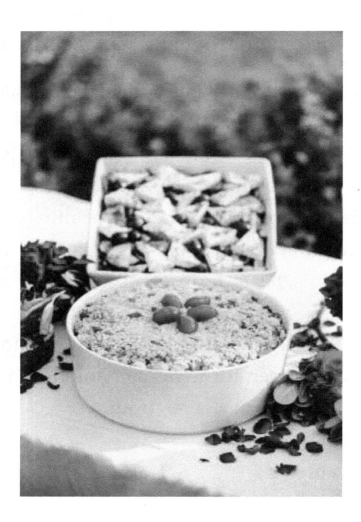

The Bottom Line

In spite of the fact that there isn't one characterized Mediterranean diet, this method of eating is for the most part wealthy in healthy plant food sources and generally lower in creature nourishments, with an emphasis on fish and fish. You can locate an entire universe of data about the Mediterranean diet on the web, and numerous extraordinary books have been expounded on it. Take a stab at go ogling "Mediterranean plans" and you will discover a huge load of extraordinary tips for heavenly suppers. By the day's end, the Mediterranean diet is inconceivably healthy and fulfilling. You will not be frustrated.

The Mediterranean diet Recipes

The following part of the book consists of the 70+ healthy and easy to make Mediterranean diet recipes which anyone can prepare at their home.

Breakfast Recipes

To follow the Mediterranean diet, you realize you ought to stack your plate with vegetables and useful for you proteins like salmon. Be that as it may, shouldn't something be said about breakfast? Natural product, dairy, and entire grains assume a major part in the diet, so there's in reality a great deal of delicious (and satisfying) breakfast alternatives to browse. Here are some delicious recipes to give you a go.

Spinach Artichoke Frittata

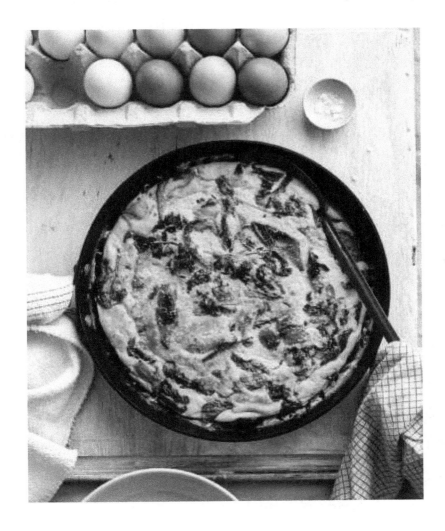

Frittatas have for quite some time been my go-to arrangement whenever I need to go through the dismal looking produce, shriveling spices, and little stubs of cheddar in my ice chest. Rarely do I make them with an arrangement up to this point.

Roused by my number one messy plunge and the warm spring climate, I concocted a frittata stacked with garlicky marinated artichoke hearts, hearty child spinach, pungent Parma, and rich harsh cream. I realized it would be acceptable, yet it blew away the entirety of my assumptions. Also, presently it's the lone frittata I need to make. In case you're not effectively all around familiar with it, you should realize that your supermarket's antipasti bar is fundamentally a secret stash of heavenly and helpful fixings.

Making a beeline for the antipasti bar is a specific must for this frittata, on the grounds that the marinated artichokes you'll discover there go about as the essential flavor promoter for your frittata. In contrast to their canned or frozen brethren, marinated artichokes are imbued with traces of garlic, spices, and appetizing olive oil that take this whenever egg dish from great to breathtaking.

Ingredients

- 10 huge eggs
- 1/2 cup full-fat harsh cream
- 1 tablespoon Dijon mustard
- 1 teaspoon fit salt
- 1/4 teaspoon newly ground dark pepper
- 1 cup ground Parmesan cheddar (around 3 ounces), separated
- 2 tablespoons olive oil
- Around 14 ounces marinated artichoke hearts, depleted, wiped off, and quartered
- 5 ounces child spinach (around 5 stuffed cups)
- 2 cloves garlic, minced

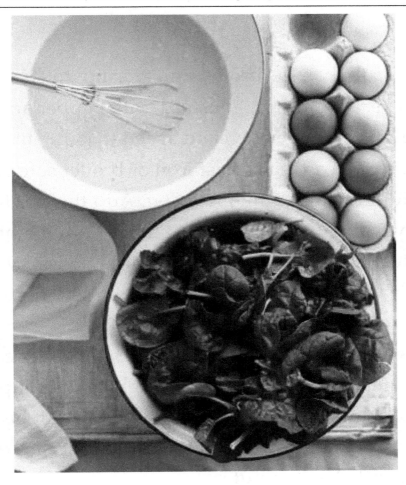

INSTRUCTIONS

- Orchestrate a rack in the broiler and warmth to 400°F.

- Spot the eggs, acrid cream, mustard, salt, pepper and 1/2 cup of the Parmesan in a huge bowl and speed to join; put in a safe spot.

- Warmth the oil in a 10-inch cast iron or broiler safe nonstick skillet over medium warmth until gleaming. Add the artichokes in a solitary layer and cook, blending at times, until daintily sautéed, 6 to 8 minutes. Add the spinach and garlic, and throw until the spinach is shriveled and practically the entirety of the fluid is vanished, around 2 minutes.

- Spread everything into an even layer. Pour the egg combination over the vegetables. Sprinkle with the excess 1/2 cup Parmesan. Slant the container to ensure the eggs settle equitably over all the vegetables. Cook undisturbed until the eggs at the edges of the dish start to set, 2 to 3 minutes.

- Prepare until the eggs are totally set, 12 to 15 minutes. To check, cut a little cut in the focal point of the frittata. In the event that crude eggs run into the cut, prepare for an additional couple of moments. Cool in the prospect minutes, at that point cut into wedges and serve warm.

1. Hearty Breakfast Fruit Salad

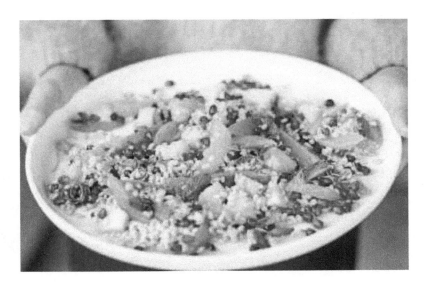

A seared grapefruit, a tasty smoothie bowl, or even a good smoothie is an enchanting method to begin quickly. In any case, some work day mornings require in excess of an organic product filled beginning, regardless of how yummy, to get your motors running and keep them running. You need something with protein and fiber, crammed with supplements; something quick that is fulfilling, energizing, and welcoming to start your motor. Here's another response to this predicament: a good entire grain and new natural product serving of mixed greens, with new spices that add measurement, and speedy sparkle of a sweet-tart dressing. It's totally made ahead and simply needs a very late throw together. This fruity tabouli is an equation, a formula outline that is so flexible you'll be having an alternate breakfast each day for quite a long time easily.

NGREDIENTS

For the grains:

- 1 cup pearl or hulled grain or any tough entire grain (see the rundown above)
- 3 cups water
- 3 tablespoons olive or vegetable oil, isolated
- 1/2 teaspoon legitimate salt
- For the natural product (see list above):
- 1/2 huge pineapple, stripped and cut into 1/2-to 2-inch lumps (2 to 2 1/2 cups)
- 6 medium tangerines or mandarins, or 5 huge oranges (around 1/2 pounds complete)
- 1/4 cups pomegranate seeds
- 1 little pack new mint

For the dressing:

- 1/3 cup nectar or another sugar (see list above)
- Juice and finely ground zing of 1 lemon (around 1/4 cup juice)
- Juice and finely ground zing of 2 limes (around 1/4 cup juice)
- 1/2 teaspoon legitimate salt
- 1/4 cup olive oil

1/4 cup toased hazelnut or nut oil

Equipment

- Estimating cups and spoons
- 2 rimmed preparing sheets
- Material paper
- Fine-network sifter
- Delicate silicone spatula

- 2 pots or 1 pan and a microwave-safe bowl
- Sharp blade
- 3 huge impenetrable holders with covers
- 2 more modest sealed shut compartments with covers
- 1 (3-cup) sealed shut compartment with a cover
- Blending bowl
- Wire whisk

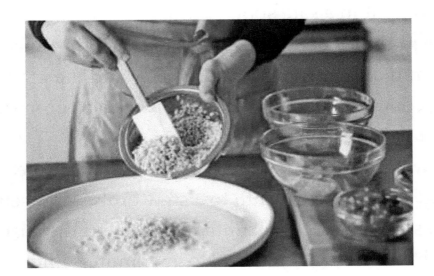

Instructions

- **Wash the grain**: Line 2 rimmed preparing sheets with material paper. Flush the grain in a sifter under virus water until the water beneath is clear, around 1 moment. Delicately shake the sifter to deplete off any overabundance water. Spot the grain on one of the readied preparing sheets and utilize a spatula to spread out the grains into a solitary layer. Let dry totally, 3 to 5 minutes.

- **Warmth the water**: Warm the water on the burner or in the microwave; put in a safe spot.

- **Toast the grain**: Heat 2 tablespoons of the oil in a medium pot over high warmth until gleaming. Cautiously add the grain and toast, blending continually, until they simply start to obscure somewhat, 1 moment to 90 seconds.

- **Add the water:** Add the warm water and salt and heat to the point of boiling. Lessen the warmth to a stew or the least setting your burner has, cover, and cook until delicate and the vast majority of the fluid has been consumed, 40 to 45 minutes. Eliminate the pot from the warmth and let stand, covered, for 10 minutes, to allow the grain to steam and wrap up engrossing the water. In the meantime, prep the natural product, mint, and dressing.

- **Set up the organic product:** Place the pineapple lumps into one of the enormous compartments. Strip and cut the tangerines, mandarins, or oranges into fragments, eliminating as a large part of the severe white substance as possible. Spot in the compartment, cover, and refrigerate. Refrigerate the pomegranate seeds independently in a covered compartment.

- **Set up the mint:** Thinly cut or mince the mint leaves then refrigerate in its own covered holder.

- **Make the dressing:** Whisk the nectar, squeeze and flavors, and salt together in a medium bowl. Sprinkle in the olive oil, at that point the nut oil, while whisking continually until consolidated. Cover and refrigerate, or refrigerate in a container.

- **Dry and cool the grain**: Transfer the cooked grain onto the second arranged preparing sheet and spread into an even layer. Let cool totally, 10 to 20 minutes. Shower the grain with the leftover 1 tablespoon of oil and blend to cover.

- **Chill the cooked grain:** Transfer the grain to a huge holder, cover, and refrigerate.

Gather the plate of mixed greens and eat: To serve, scoop 2/3 cup of the grain into each bowl. Add around 6 bits of pineapple, 10 to 12 orange portions, and 1/4 cup pomegranate seeds into each bowl. Add 1 to 2 tablespoons of the mint and 2 to 3 tablespoons of the dressing to each bowl (re-whisk the dressing if necessary). Mix to blend and cover with the dressing.

2. The Best Shakshuka

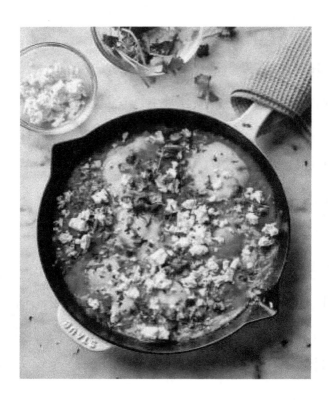

- Shakshuka is a one-skillet dish of eggs poached in fragrant, spiced pureed tomatoes. In North Africa, Israel, and different pieces of the Middle East where it's discovered, it's frequently served for breakfast however it's generous enough to be delighted in any season of day, particularly when presented with pita or other bread to swipe up the sassy blend. It tends to be set up in various manners, and each form varies in its blend of flavors and aromatics. And keeping in mind that the tomato-based rendition is generally normal, there are numerous other flavorful translations (green shakshuka, for instance, is additionally worth difficult).

- In the event that you generally request shakshuka at your number one early lunch spot yet you've never attempted to make the dish at home, this formula is the absolute best spot to begin. The Middle Eastern egg dish has gotten fiercely well known, all things considered: It's incredibly soothing and pretty darn simple to make at home. Whenever you've taken in the couple of keys to progress, which we've laid out beneath, you'll be exceptional to make some extraordinary shakshuka at whatever point you need, regardless of whether for informal breakfast or a simple weeknight supper.

INGREDIENTS

- 1 (28-ounce) can entire stripped tomatoes
- 2 tablespoons olive oil
- 1 little yellow onion, finely hacked
- 2 tablespoons tomato glue
- 1 tablespoon harissa
- 3 cloves garlic, minced
- 1 teaspoon ground cumin
- 1/2 teaspoon genuine salt
- 6 huge eggs
- 1/4 cup approximately stuffed slashed new cilantro leaves and delicate stems
- 2 ounces feta cheddar, disintegrated (around 1/2 cup, discretionary)

    Hard bread or pita, for serving (discretionary)

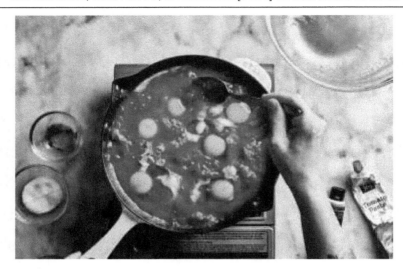

- **INSTRUCTIONS**
- Pulverize the tomatoes. Pour the tomatoes and their juices into a huge bowl. Cautiously squash with your hands into scaled down pieces; put in a safe spot.
- Sauté the aromatics. Warmth the oil in a 10-or 12-inch skillet over medium warmth until shining. Add the onion and sauté until clear and mellowed, 5 to 6 minutes. Add the tomato glue, harissa, garlic, cumin, and salt, and sauté until fragrant, around 1 moment.
- Stew the pureed tomatoes for 10 minutes. Add the tomatoes and bring to a stew. Stew delicately until the sauce has thickened marginally, around 10 minutes.
- Break the eggs into the sauce. Eliminate the skillet from the warmth. Make 6 little wells in the sauce. Break an egg into each well.
- Spoon some sauce over the egg whites. Delicately spoon a touch of sauce over the egg whites, leaving the yolks uncovered (this will help the whites cook quicker so they set before the yolks). Cover and return the skillet to medium-low warmth.
- Cook the eggs 8 to 12 minutes. Cook, turning the dish depending on the situation with the goal that the eggs cook uniformly, until the whites are set and the yolks are to your ideal doneness, 8 to 12 minutes (keep an eye on it a couple of times). The eggs should in any case wiggle in the focuses when you delicately shake the skillet.
- Get done with cilantro and cheddar. Eliminate from the warmth. Sprinkle with the cilantro and feta, if utilizing, and present with bread or pita whenever wanted.

Balsamic Berries with Honey Yogurt

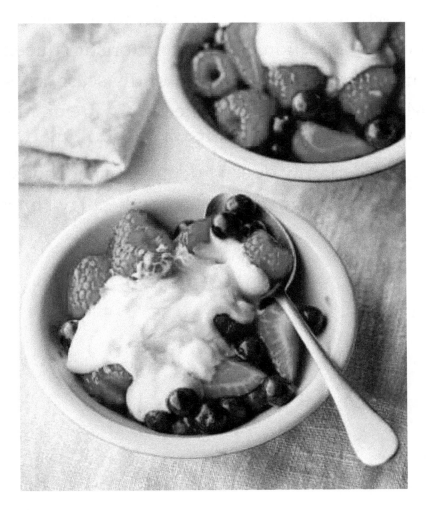

At the point when new berries are at their pinnacle mid-summer, I can't resist the urge to eat my weight in them. I sprinkle them onto my morning oats, eat them insane noontime, and appreciate them as a sweet yet healthy treat after supper. This snappy formula accepts the delicious summer leafy foods them into a quick and extravagant treat surprisingly fast. You may as of now have the ingredients in your kitchen at the present time, which implies this could be pastry tonight.t may appear to be strange to throw berries in vinegar for dessert, yet in the event that you've at any point attempted this mix, you realize how well it works. Balsamic vinegar, while tart, has a characteristic pleasantness to it.

At the point when showered over strawberries, blueberries, and raspberries, it draws a portion of the characteristic squeezes and sugars out of the natural product to make profoundly seasoned syrup for them to swim in. Much the same as that, the berries are an ideal method to cover off a dinner, however completing them with a spot of nectar improved yogurt certainly doesn't do any harm. Choose entire milk plain Greek yogurt for the smoothest lavishness.

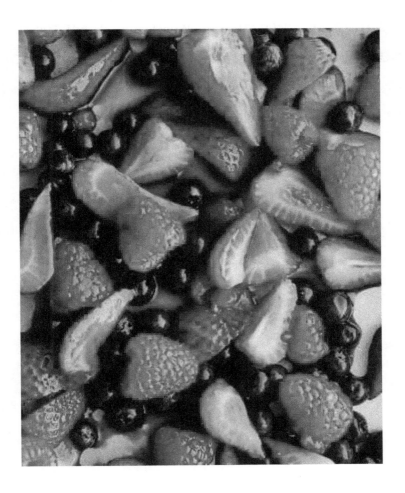

INGREDIENTS

- 8 ounces strawberries, hulled and divided, or quartered if exceptionally enormous (around 1/2 cups)
- 1 cup blueberries
- 1 cup raspberries
- 1 tablespoon balsamic vinegar
- 2/3 cup entire milk plain Greek yogurt
- 2 teaspoons nectar

INSTRUCTIONS

Throw the strawberries, blueberries, and raspberries with the balsamic vinegar in an enormous bowl. Let it sit for 10 minutes. Mix the yogurt and nectar together in a little bowl. Split the berries between serving bowls or glasses and top each with a touch of nectar yogurt.

3. Caprese Avocado Toast

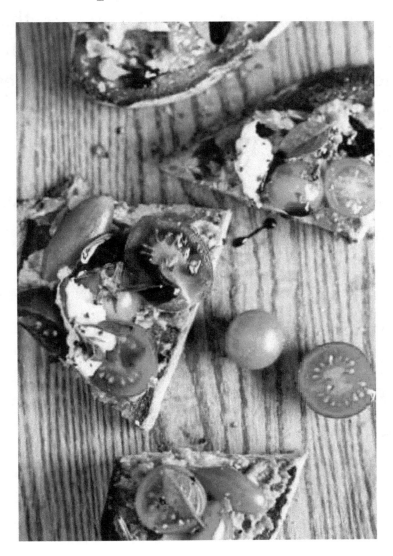

- With regards to avocado toast, the best cuts work out positively past two ingredients. On the off chance that you require additional verification, let us present this caprese avocado toast. All the segments of a caprese serving of mixed greens from the ready tomatoes and the smooth mozzarella to the new basil and the tart balsamic coating are an old buddy to the cool avocado. In the event that there was ever an illustration of when the entire is superior to the amount of its parts (and we're discussing powerful parts!), caprese avocado toast nails it on the head.

- While fat, round tomatoes and thick cuts of mozzarella are the stars of caprese serving of mixed greens, think more modest with regards to avocado toast. Stick with reduced down ingredients, similar to grape or cherry tomatoes and pearl-sized bundles of mozzarella.

INGREDIENTS

- 2 cuts generous sandwich bread, for example, worker bread, sourdough, entire wheat or multi-grain
- 1 medium avocado, split and pit eliminated
- 8 grape tomatoes, split
- 2 ounces new ciliegine or scaled down mozzarella balls (around 12)
- 4 huge new basil leaves, torn

2 tablespoons balsamic coating

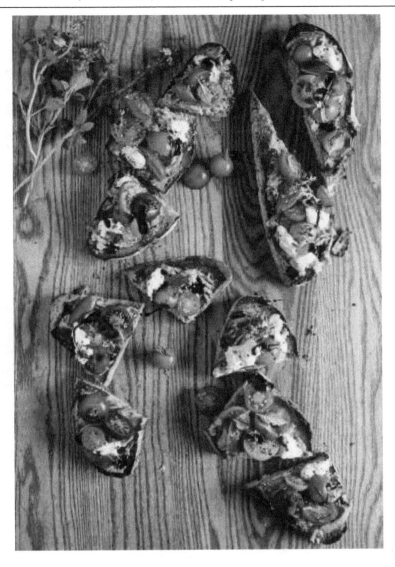

INSTRUCTIONS

Toast the bread. While the bread is toasting, crush the avocado in a little bowl.

Spread the crushed avocado over the toast. Top each cut with tomatoes, mozzarella balls, and basil leaves, at that point sprinkle with balsamic coating. Serve right away

Spinach Feta Breakfast Wraps

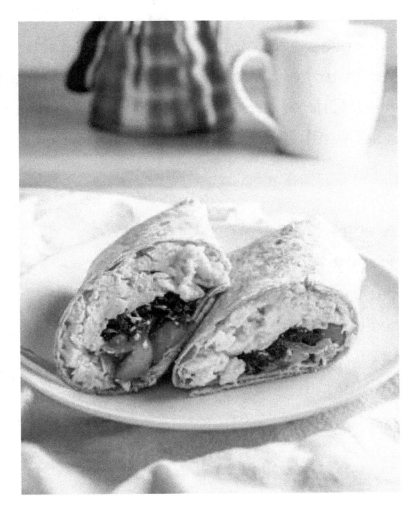

Pre-winter, when fresh mornings cause me to disregard chilled for the time being oats and smoothies, and rather push warm morning meals to the front of my psyche. The lone test is finding warm morning meals that are still speedy enough to make on occupied fall mornings. Enter these cooler well-disposed breakfast wraps.

Following these tips for freezing burritos, I made veggie lover wraps loaded up with eggs, tomatoes, spinach, and feta that are prepared to microwave in the first part of the day. Skipping breakfast at Starbucks is much simpler when I can have this on my plate in just two minutes.

You could dress these wraps up with any fillings you'd like, yet I love this five-fixing variant enlivened by the wraps at Starbucks. This hits all the pivotal flavor focuses — exquisite eggs and spinach, pleasantly acidic tomatoes, and pungent feta cheddar — while remaining healthfully balanced. One of these wraps in addition to a hot mug of espresso, and I'm set until at any rate early afternoon.

INGREDIENTS

- 10 enormous eggs
- 1/2 pound (around 5 cups) infant spinach
- 4 entire wheat tortillas (around 9 creeps in width, burrito-sized)
- 1/2 16 ounces cherry or grape tomatoes, divided
- 4 ounces feta cheddar, disintegrated
- Margarine or olive oil
- Salt
- Pepper

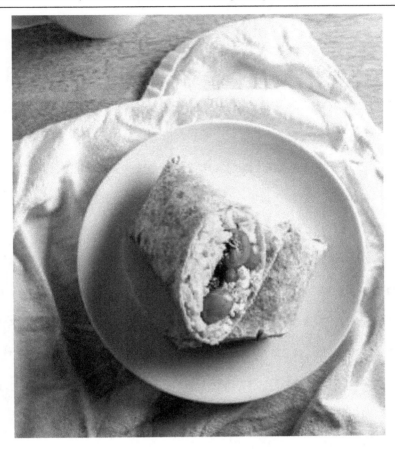

INSTRUCTIONS

- In a huge bowl, whisk the eggs until the whites and yolks are totally joined. Spot an enormous skillet over medium warmth and add sufficient spread or olive oil to cover the base. At the point when the spread is liquefied or the oil is hot, pour in the eggs and mix infrequently until the eggs are cooked. Mix when there's no other option of salt and a liberal measure of dark pepper, at that point move to a huge plate to cool to room temperature.

- Wash or wipe down the skillet, place it back over medium warmth, and add another part of margarine or oil. Add the spinach and cook, blending frequently, until the spinach is simply shriveled. Spread the cooked spinach on another enormous plate to cool to room temperature.

- Organize a tortilla on a work surface. Add about a quarter every one of the eggs, spinach, tomatoes, and feta down the center of the tortilla and firmly wrap (perceive How to Wrap a Burrito). Rehash with the leftover three tortillas. Spot a couple envelops by a gallon zip-top pack and freeze until prepared to eat. In the event that freezing for over seven days, wrap the burritos in aluminum foil to forestall cooler consume. To warm, microwave on high for 2 minutes.

- Easy Homemade Muesli

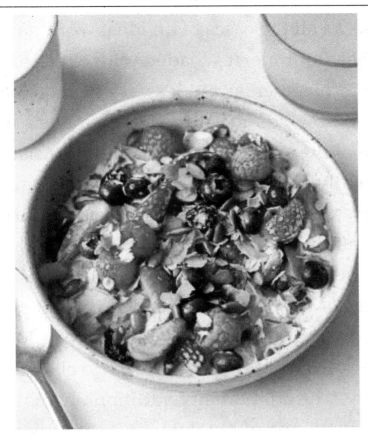

- Muesli began in Switzerland by a doctor named Maximilian Bircher-Benner. His form, regularly alluded to as "Bircher muesli," comprised of whole oats, ground apples, and hacked nuts blended in with lemon squeeze, water, and improved consolidated milk. Today, muesli all the more regularly alludes to a blend of moved oats, nuts, seeds, and dried organic product. Consider it a better, low-sugar option in contrast to granola. Since muesli isn't prepared, there's no sugar or oil expected to tie the ingredients together despite the fact that I do get a kick out of the chance to toast the grains, nuts, and seeds before they're combined as one to draw out their flavors. It's additionally ideal to throw the grain with a warm flavor (like cinnamon, nutmeg, cardamom, cloves, or ginger) prior to toasting.

- Muesli checks all the cases of an ideal work day breakfast. You can make it ahead of time; it's loaded with entire grains, fiber, protein, and cell reinforcements; and it's very flexible, both by the way you cause it and how you to eat it. I like to make a major clump over the course of the end of the week to last consistently, which fundamentally accelerates my work day morning schedule. It's hot, nutty, chewy, and really fulfilling at last, a morning meal that can hold me until lunch.....Muesli can likewise be appreciated like cereal (on the off chance that I eat it along these lines, I top it with cut bananas or new berries), blended into yogurt, or heated up with milk or water and eaten like oats. To hold my morning meal routine back from feeling static, I like to change things up consistently. The adaptability additionally makes this a morning meal dish every one of my flat mates can concur on, in light of the fact that we've all discovered our #1 method to set it up. On the off chance that you do favor your morning meal on the better side, any of these arrangements can be done with a sprinkle of nectar or maple syrup, in spite of the fact that I locate a garnish of new organic product gives the perfect measure of pleasantness.

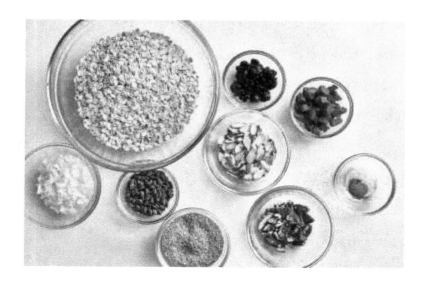

INGREDIENTS

- 3 1/2 cups moved oats
- 1/2 cup wheat grain
- 1/2 teaspoon legitimate salt
- 1/2 teaspoon ground cinnamon
- 1/2 cup cut almonds
- 1/4 cup crude walnuts, coarsely cleaved
- 1/4 cup crude pepitas (shelled pumpkin seeds)
- 1/2 cup unsweetened coconut chips
- 1/4 cup dried apricots, coarsely cleaved
- 1/4 cup dried cherries

INSTRUCTIONS

- Toast the grains, nuts, and seeds. Organize 2 racks to partition the stove into thirds and warmth to 350°F. Spot the oats, wheat grain, salt, and cinnamon on a rimmed preparing sheet; throw to join; and spread into an even layer. Spot the almonds, walnuts, and pepitas on a second rimmed heating sheet; throw to consolidate; and spread into an even layer. Move both preparing sheets to stove, setting oats on top rack and nuts on base. Prepare until nuts are fragrant, 10 to 12 minutes.
- Add the coconut. Eliminate the heating sheet with the nuts and put aside to cool. Sprinkle the coconut over the oats, get back to the upper rack, and prepare until the coconut is brilliant earthy colored, around 5 minutes more. Eliminate from broiler and put aside to cool, around 10 minutes.

- Move to an enormous bowl. Move the substance of both preparing sheets to an enormous bowl.

- Add the dried organic product. Add the apricots and cherries and throw to consolidate.

- Move to an impermeable compartment. Muesli can be put away in a hermetically sealed compartment at room temperature for as long as multi month.

- Appreciate as wanted. Appreciate as oats, grain, short-term oats, or with yogurt, finished off with new leafy foods sprinkle of nectar or maple syrup, whenever wanted.

4. Kale and Goat Cheese Frittata Cups

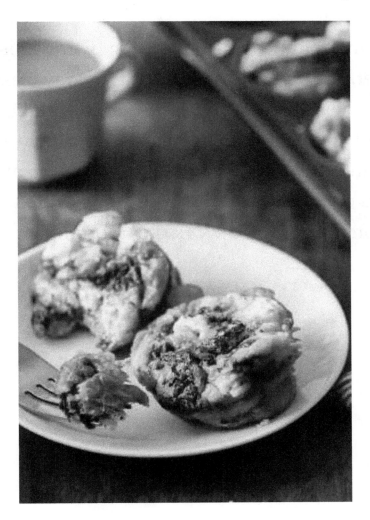

Frittatas are decent on the grounds that they're basic, and these frittata cups are easy to the point that they can sensibly advance into the work day arrangement.

While they are intended to be served warm, they're really magnificent room temperature or even cool, making them an incredible in and out lunch choice too. Furthermore, this formula is adaptable. Try not to like kale? Substitute an alternate verdant green. Have broccoli you need to go through? Cleave it up and toss it in. Lean toward Parmesan to goat cheddar? Forget about it. You can test here and discover an adaptation of this formula that suits your own taste.

In our home, frittatas, the Italian egg dish that is frequently made in a skillet, are typically saved for a Sunday clear out-the-cooler evening. They're easy to put together, fulfilling, and you can utilize practically any vegetable or cheddar you have available. In any case, of late, they've been advancing onto the morning meal table. All things considered, to be honest, I've been doing a compact adaptation for occupied work day mornings.

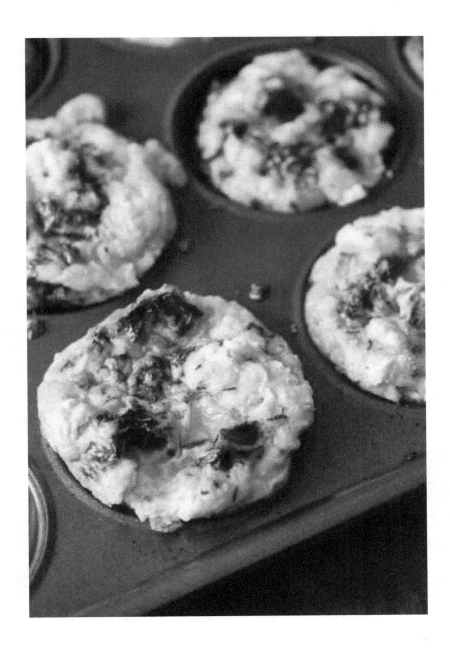

INGREDIENTS

2 cups hacked lacinato kale

- 1 garlic clove, daintily cut

- 3 tablespoons olive oil
- 1/4 teaspoon red pepper pieces
- 8 enormous eggs
- 1/4 teaspoon salt
- Run ground dark pepper
- 1/2 teaspoon dried thyme
- 1/4 cup goat cheddar, disintegrated

INSTRUCTIONS

- Preheat the broiler to 350°F. To get 2 cups kale, eliminate the leaves from the kale ribs. Wash and dry the leaves and cut them into 1/2-inch-wide strips.
- In a 10-inch nonstick skillet, cook the garlic in 1 tablespoon of oil over medium-high warmth for 30 seconds. Add the kale and red pepper chips and cook until withered, 1 to 2 minutes.
- In a medium bowl, beat the eggs with the salt and pepper. Add the kale and thyme to the egg blend.
- Utilizing a 12-cup biscuit tin, utilize the excess 2 tablespoons of oil to oil 8 of the cups (you may likewise utilize margarine or nonstick splash on the off chance that you'd like). Sprinkle the tops with goat cheddar. Prepare until they are set in the middle, around 25 to 30 minutes.
- Frittata is best eaten warm from the stove or inside the following day, yet extras can be kept refrigerated and warmed for as long as seven days.

- ## Avocado and Egg Breakfast Pizza

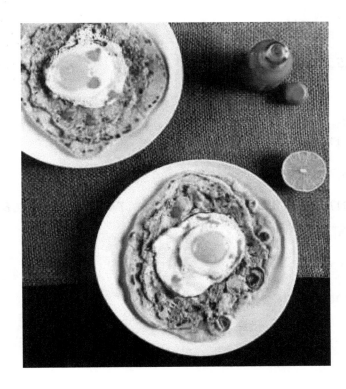

- Presumably don't need to reveal to you that consolidating three of the world's most prominent nourishments gives you one fine breakfast: a warm round of chewy hull finished off with a splendid, cilantro-dotted avocado crush, and the ideal sloppy egg.

- I've generally had breakfast; however for a long time I stayed alive on cereal with milk, or toast with margarine and jam straightforward, carb-y suppers that normally left me a few hours after the fact. My propensities have changed and now my morning meals consistently incorporate an aiding of protein and fat alongside my carbs, which help to keep me fulfilled until noon. Avocados and eggs frequently show up, however not ordinarily on a similar plate. That is the thing that makes this formula exceptional.

INGREDIENTS

1 huge Hass avocado

- 1 tablespoon finely slashed cilantro
- 1/2 teaspoons lime juice
- 1/8 teaspoon salt
- 1/2 pound pizza batter, hand crafted or locally acquired (see Recipe Note)
- 4 huge eggs
- 1 tablespoon vegetable oil

Hot sauce, for serving (discretionary)

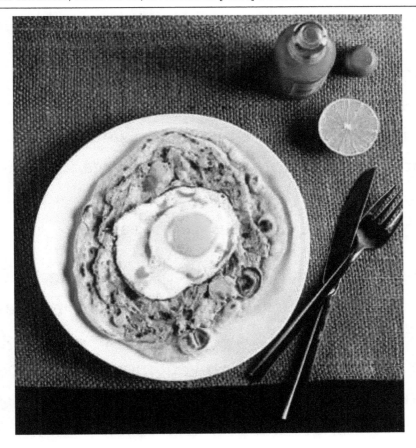

INSTRUCTIONS

Cut the avocado down the middle the long way, eliminate the pit and, with a huge spoon, scoop the tissue into a medium bowl. Add the cilantro, lime squeeze and salt. Crush with a fork until smooth, with a couple of pieces of avocado. Taste and change preparing. (Contingent upon the size of your avocado, you may require more salt or lime juice.) Set aside.

- Separation the mixture into 4 equivalent pieces. On an all-around floured cutting board, fold each piece into a dainty 6-inch circle. (In the event that the mixture continues to spring back as you move it, let it rest for a couple of moments to loosen up the gluten and attempt once more.)

- Warmth an all-around prepared cast iron skillet (see Recipe Note) over medium-high warmth until hot. Spot one of the mixture circles in the focal point of the skillet. Cook for 1 to 2 minutes, until the underside is sautéed and the top surface is bubbly. Flip and cook opposite side until seared, pushing down with a spatula if the batter puffs up off the lower part of the skillet. It could be burned in spots, which is fine. Move to a plate and rehash with outstanding batter circles.

- Spread 1/4 of the avocado combination onto each cooked piece of mixture.

- Warmth the oil in a skillet over medium warmth. (In the event that utilizing a similar skillet you utilized for the mixture, first let it cool somewhat and clear out any consumed flour that might be adhering to it.) Fry eggs to wanted doneness and spot everyone on top of a pizza. Serve quickly, with or without a sprinkle of hot sauce.

5. Smashed Egg Toasts with Herby Lemon   Yogurt

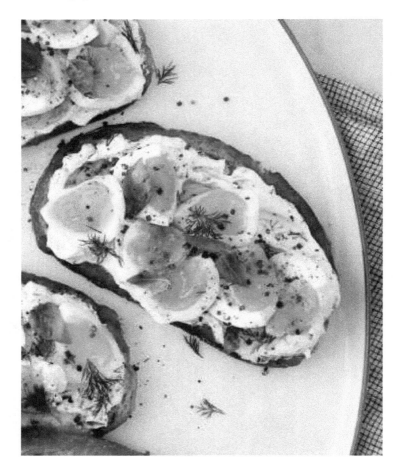

A completely cooked egg on hot buttered toast is, as far as I might be concerned, the stuff of dreams. Truth be told, I've basically gotten a specialist at hoisting the egg-on-toast combo. From frog in-the-opening to extravagant avocado toast and so on, I've made it.

My most recent redesign includes another most loved breakfast thing: yogurt! You'll begin by stirring up a flavorful Greek yogurt spread that is loaded with lemon and garlic, at that point spread it over the toast. Gently crush delicate bubbled eggs on top to make scraggly little pieces — they'll blend in with the yogurt and make an egg serving of mixed greens like combination that is smooth and rich. A light shower of olive oil and liberal topping of spices balance the entire thing, and unexpectedly the unassuming egg toast is a finished (and rich!) feast.

INGREDIENTS

- 8 huge eggs
- 1 clove garlic
- 1 medium lemon
- 2 tablespoons finely slashed new basil leaves, in addition to additional for embellish
- 2 tablespoons finely slashed new dill, in addition to additional for embellish
- 2 tablespoons finely hacked new chives, in addition to additional for embellish
- 2 cups plain Greek yogurt
- 2 tablespoons extra-virgin olive oil, in addition to additional for showering
- 3/4 teaspoon legitimate salt, in addition to additional for sprinkling
- 1/2 teaspoon newly ground dark pepper, in addition to additional for sprinkling
- 4 huge cuts country or sourdough bread (around 1-inch thick)

4 tablespoons unsalted spread, separated

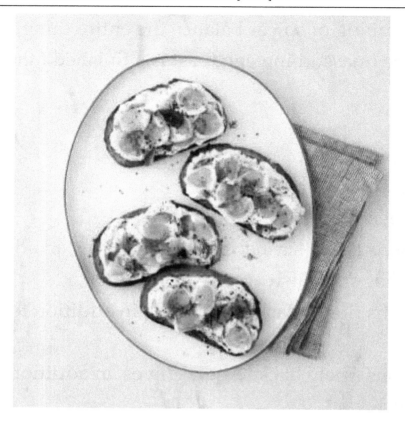

INSTRUCTIONS

- Fill an enormous pot with around 5 creeps of water and bring to a turning bubble over high warmth; fill a huge bowl with cold water and ice. Lower the warmth until the water is at a quick stew. Tenderly lower 8 enormous eggs into the water each in turn. Bubble for precisely 6 minutes and 30 seconds. Utilizing an opened spoon, move the eggs to the ice shower. Let sit in the ice shower for 2 minutes, at that point strip the eggs under running water and put them in a safe spot.

- Set up the accompanying, adding them to a medium bowl: Mince 1 garlic clove. Finely grind the zing 1 medium lemon; at that point squeeze the lemon. Finely hack until you have 2 tablespoons new basil leaves, 2 tablespoons new dill, and 2 tablespoons new chives. Add 2 cups Greek yogurt, 2 tablespoons extra-virgin olive oil, 3/4 teaspoon fit salt, and 1/2 teaspoon dark pepper. Mix to consolidate.

- Cut 4 (1-inch thick) cuts dried up bread. Dissolve 2 tablespoons unsalted spread in an enormous skillet over medium warmth. Add 2 of the cuts and cook until brilliant earthy colored and fresh, around 2 minutes for each side. Move to a huge platter. Rehash with the excess 2 tablespoons unsalted margarine and bread.

Spread the yogurt blend on the bread; at that point top each toast with 2 of the eggs. Utilizing the rear of a spoon, delicately crush the eggs. Sprinkle with more genuine salt, dark pepper, and spices, and shower with more olive oil.

Lunch Recipes

Breakfast may be the main supper of the day, yet lunch is regularly the most ignored. Between picking the most straightforward alternative (cold extras!) and making the time amidst telecommuting (and possibly additionally "educating" kids), it's no big surprise we need that evening mug of espresso so seriously. In spite of your opinion, eating a sound, delightful lunch each day doesn't mean you need to commit your whole Sunday to supper prep, and we're here to demonstrate it. Continue to peruse for brisk lunch plans you can make very quickly.

Chickpea Pancakes With Greens and Cheese

These messy, green-y, and absolutely fulfilling chickpea hotcakes were roused by Healthyish benefactor Aliza Abarbanel's #1 work-from-home solace lunch. "I've filled these hotcakes with pretty much every extra in the cooler, from cooked greens to broiled mushrooms to marinated lentils, however melty cheddar stays a consistent," she says. Sans gluten and loaded with protein, chickpea flour flapjacks come in numerous varieties across the world, from Indian besan chilla to French socca to Italian farinata. In the event that you don't feel like or have the opportunity to make hotcake player during your mid-day break (however we energetically suggest it!) huge flour or alt-flour tortillas work superbly as a substitute; simply crease the cooked greens and cheddar inside the tortillas and warmth straightforwardly in the skillet to soften the cheddar.

Fixings

- 2 SERVINGS
- ½ cup chickpea flour
- 3 Tbsp. additionally 4 tsp. olive oil, separated
- Fit salt
- ½ medium red onion, meagerly cut
- 4 garlic cloves, crushed
- 1 cup brussels sprouts, meagerly cut
- little pack Tuscan kale or other kale, ribs and stems eliminated, meagerly cut

- tsp. hot sauce, in addition to additional for serving
- oz. sharp cheddar, coarsely ground
- Plain yogurt (for serving)

Arrangement

Stage 1

Preheat stove to 350°. Whisk chickpea flour and ½ cup in addition to 2 Tbsp. cold water in a little bowl. Rush in 1 Tbsp. oil and a touch of salt. Let sit at any rate 10 minutes and as long as 1 hour to permit flour to hydrate.

Stage 2

In the interim, heat 2 Tbsp. oil in a huge nonstick skillet over medium-high. Add onion, garlic, and brussels sprouts; cook, throwing sporadically, until mollified and softly seared, around 3 minutes. Add kale and cook, throwing frequently, until delicate, around 3 minutes. Add 2 tsp. hot sauce, season with salt, and throw well. Move to a medium bowl; clear out skillet.

Stage 3

Twirl 1 tsp. oil in skillet to cover; heat over medium-high. Empty ¼ cup hitter into focus of skillet and twirl to shape a dainty 6"– 7"-measurement flapjack. Cook until very much sautéed under and fresh around edges, around 2 minutes. Flip hotcake and cook just until second side is gently carmelized, around 1 moment. Move to a rimmed heating sheet. Rehash measure with residual player and 3 tsp. oil to make 4 aggregate. Split vegetables between 2 flapjacks and top with cheddar and staying 2 hotcakes. Heat until cheddar is liquefied, 6–8 minutes. Serve finished off with yogurt and more hot sauce.

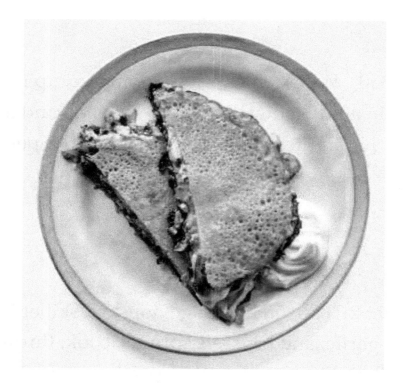

Lunch Nachos With Spiced Cauliflower

Test Kitchen chief Chris Morocco depends on some adaptation of these lunch nachos in any event once every week as he conceptualizes what to take care of his two little youngsters. It's awesome to submit the recipe to memory: a pack of chips, a container of refried beans, perhaps some extra meat or simmered veg from the prior night, destroyed cheddar, and some sort of immediately cooked, spiced veg like cauliflower or brussels sprouts. It's a lightning-quick lunch (or supper) that can be changed to suit anybody's inclinations.

Fixings

2 SERVINGS

- 1 cup daintily cut radishes, red onion, cabbage, carrots, or other firm vegetable
- ½ cup prepared rice vinegar
- 3 Tbsp. extra-virgin olive oil, partitioned
- 2 garlic cloves, crushed
- ½ little head of cauliflower, divided through stem end, meagerly cut
- 1 tsp. ground coriander
- 1 tsp. ground cumin
- 1 tsp. paprika
- Genuine salt
- 8 oz. tortilla chips
- 1 cup refried beans (like Amy's)

- 8 oz. sharp cheddar, coarsely ground
- Cleaved avocado, cilantro leaves with delicate stems, and plain yogurt (for serving)

Readiness

Stage 1

Throw radishes and vinegar in a little bowl to consolidate; put in a safe spot.

Stage 2

Preheat stove to 400°. Warmth 2 Tbsp. oil in a huge skillet over medium-high. Cook garlic, throwing frequently, until brilliant around edges, around 2 minutes. Add cauliflower; cook, undisturbed, until brilliant earthy colored under, around 3 minutes. Throw, at that point keep on cooking, throwing infrequently, until seared all finished and fresh delicate, around 3 minutes more. Add coriander, cumin, paprika, and staying 1 Tbsp. oil. Cook, throwing, until fragrant, around 1 moment; season with salt.

Stage 3

Spread portion of chips on a little rimmed preparing sheet. Organize half of cauliflower on top. Bit half of beans over, at that point sprinkle with half of cheddar. Rehash layers once again. Prepare until cheddar is softened, 10–12 minutes. Top with depleted radishes, avocado, cilantro, and yogurt.

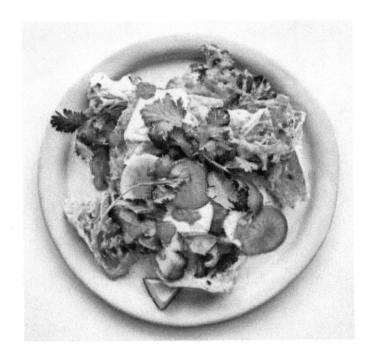

Broccoli Melts

Here's a working-from-home lunch that's quick enough to make between Zooms and will send you well on your way to meeting your daily veg quota. While there's something satisfying about the airy crustiness of a baguette, halved ciabatta rolls or slices of sourdough or whole wheat bread would work just as well.

Ingredients

2 SERVINGS

- 1small shallot or ¼ red onion, thinly sliced
- 1 Tbsp. plus 1½ tsp. sherry vinegar or red wine vinegar
- Pinch of sugar
- Kosher salt, freshly ground pepper
- 1small head of broccoli (8–10 oz.)
- 3Tbsp. extra-virgin olive oil
- 1garlic clove
- 2
- Tbsp. mayonnaise
- 1 tsp. hot chili sauce (such as Sriracha)
- 2 6" pieces baguette, halved lengthwise
- 4 slices sharp cheddar

Preparation

Step 1

Heat broiler. Combine shallot, vinegar, sugar, and a pinch of salt and pepper in a small bowl. Stir to combine; set aside.

Step 2

Trim and peel broccoli stem. Remove stem from crown and finely chop. Cut crown into florets, then coarsely chop into bite-size pieces.

Step 3

Heat oil in a large ovenproof skillet over medium-high. Add broccoli; season with salt. Cook, stirring occasionally, until browned in spots, about 3 minutes. Reduce heat to medium, add ¼ cup water, and cover. Cook until tender, about 2 minutes. Reduce heat to low and uncover. Grate in garlic; add reserved shallot mixture. Cook, stirring, until vinegar is mostly evaporated, about 15 seconds. Transfer to a bowl. Reserve skillet.

Step 4

Mix mayonnaise and chili sauce in a small bowl. Taste and add more chili sauce if desired.

Step 5

Broil bread, cut side up, in reserved skillet until lightly toasted, about 1 minute (watch carefully!). Remove from oven and spread mayo mixture over. Spoon broccoli mixture on top, going all the way to the edges (don't be afraid to pile it on). Drape a slice of cheese over (tear in half if needed).

Step 6

Broil, watching carefully, until cheese is bubbling and browned, about 3 minutes. Season with pepper.

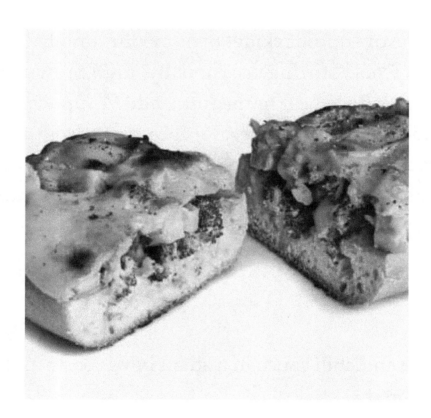

Gyeran Mari

Gourmet expert Susan Kim offers Korean to-go lunch boxes loaded up with wonderfully arranged vegetables and different banchan, or little side dishes, through her NYC-based spring up Eat Doshi. We were so fascinated of these lovely doshirak that we requested that Kim show us how to reproduce a home-cooked adaptation that incorporates these appetizing moved egg omelet cuts loaded up with toasted kelp snacks and a mysterious fixing: Parm shavings. They're similarly acceptable delighted in all alone as a little bite, as a side dish to a bigger feast, or cut and presented with a bowl of rice. Kim utilizes sheets of toasted kelp snacks from brands like Seasnax or gimMe, which come pre-prepared with sesame oil and salt. Get the formula for the celery and turnip pickles, likewise highlighted in the container.

Fixings

- 2 - 4 SERVINGS
- 5 enormous eggs
- 2 Tbsp. mirin
- ½ tsp. white or customary soy sauce
- ½ tsp. genuine salt
- 1 Tbsp. vegetable oil
- 2 oz. Parmesan, shaved with a vegetable peeler
- 6 prepared toasted ocean growth snacks

Readiness

Stage 1

Whisk eggs, mirin, soy sauce, and salt in a 2-cup estimating glass. Warmth oil in a medium nonstick skillet over medium-low. Pour in 33% of egg blend, pivoting skillet to equally circulate. Cook until egg is generally cooked, around 1 moment. Dissipate 33% of Parmesan over and shingle 2 kelp snacks vertically down the middle. Utilizing an elastic spatula and beginning from one side, overlap egg over-top itself to move up firmly; push aside. Rehash cooking measure with half of outstanding egg combination, Parmesan, and ocean growth snacks, at that point flip existing egg turn over onto level egg and move up once more. Rehash once again with residual fixings. Move gyeran mari to a plate and let cool 5 minutes. Cut into ½"- thick pieces.

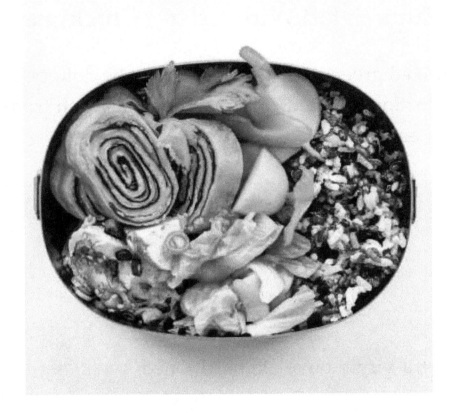

Tuna Salad With Crispy Chickpeas

Fish plate of mixed greens merits more than to be dolloped on dressed greens for lunch. Some seared chickpeas and the mash from endive improve things enormously.

Fixings

2 SERVINGS

- 5 Tbsp. extra-virgin olive oil, partitioned
- 1 15-oz. can chickpeas, flushed, wiped off
- Genuine salt
- 1 little shallot, finely cleaved
- 2 Tbsp. mayonnaise
- 1Tbsp. Dijon mustard
- 1 Tbsp. red wine vinegar
- Newly ground dark pepper
- 1 5-oz. can water-stuffed fish, depleted
- 3 red or other endive, split transversely, leaves isolated
- ½ cup parsley leaves
- 2 Tbsp. (stacking) cut salted chiles
- ½ lemon

Readiness

Stage 1

Warmth 3 Tbsp. oil in an enormous skillet over medium-high. Cook chickpeas, throwing sometimes, until fresh and brilliant earthy colored, 6–8 minutes. Season with salt and let cool.

Stage 2

Whisk shallot, mayonnaise, mustard, and vinegar in a huge bowl; season dressing with salt and pepper. Blend in fish, saying a final farewell to a fork. Add chickpeas, endive, parsley, and salted chiles. Finely grind zing from lemon over, at that point press in juice. Pour in excess 2 Tbsp. oil and throw to consolidate. Taste and season with more salt if necessary.

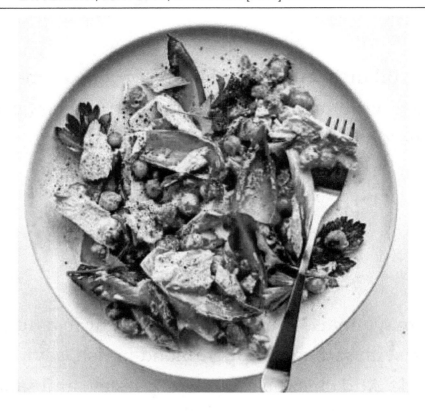

Dinner Recipes

What would it be advisable for me to make for supper around evening time that is EASY? What are some acceptable, solid meals? Could I simply pay somebody to think of a simple supper thought for me? We're food bloggers—we in a real sense cook supper professionally—and these inquiries actually frequent us now and again. Remaining there, gazing into the ice chest, considering what you can prepare this evening that everybody will happily eat and that will not require a zillion hours—definitely, we've been there! For you (and for ourselves!) we've assembled this rundown of the 60 BEST, simple supper plans we have. They're everywhere—some are solid plans, some are somewhat more liberal, some are vegan plans, some are about a major piece of protein—yet they're brought together by their effortlessness. So here you have it! Our closest to perfect, simple suppers—across the board place.

- Broccoli Pesto Pasta. To make broccoli pesto, broccoli florets are whizzed right into the pesto sauce itself, adding an even more vibrant punch of emerald green to the sauce as well as a seriously healthy boost.

- Baked Salmon with Grapefruit Salad. Moist, flaky, melt-in-your-mouth salmon perfection. This is the easy salmon recipe you've been waiting for. Oh, and did we mention it cooks in just 15 minutes?

- Lemon Chicken. This easy recipe shines with a sunny, lemony zing. Garlic and herbs—plus a glut of white wine—mean that juicy, tender chicken breasts are as delicious as they are healthy.

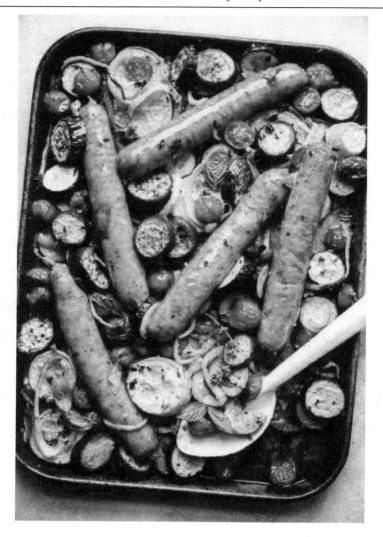

Ratatouille Sheet Pan Dinner With Sausage.

While ratatouille is delicious served all on its own, we've added sausage to the mix to take this healthy sheet pan dinner to new heights.

Salmon en Papillote.

 Who knew that such an elegant meal could be so very easy.

Instant Pot Chicken Marinara With Polenta.

Our simple equation for this easy, satisfying dinner goes something like this: chicken thighs + a jar of marinara sauce = dinner's done.

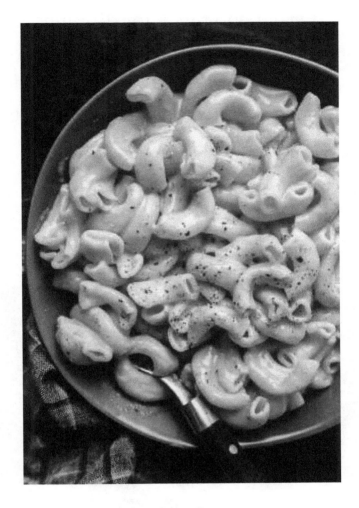

Best, Easy Dinner Recipes For A Family

- Sheet Pan Olive Bar Chicken. Full of rich flavors, almost NO prep, and using only one pan, this dish is destined to become a new favorite.
- Five Spice Chicken Sheet Pan Dinner. Chicken thighs and cabbage get a little dose of flavor from Chinese five spice, and a little oven time on a sheet pan and boom! Dinner's done.
- Sheet Pan Quesadilla with Jalapeño Ranch. Stuffed with cheese and avocado, this giant, melty, upgraded cheese sheet pan

quesadilla is good on its own, but we take it over the top with a side of homemade jalapeño ranch for dipping.

- <u>Instant Pot Mac and Cheese</u>. What's easier — and way better — than instant mac and cheese? Rich, creamy, homemade *Instant Pot* mac and cheese! Why? Because it takes about 5 minutes start-to-finish.

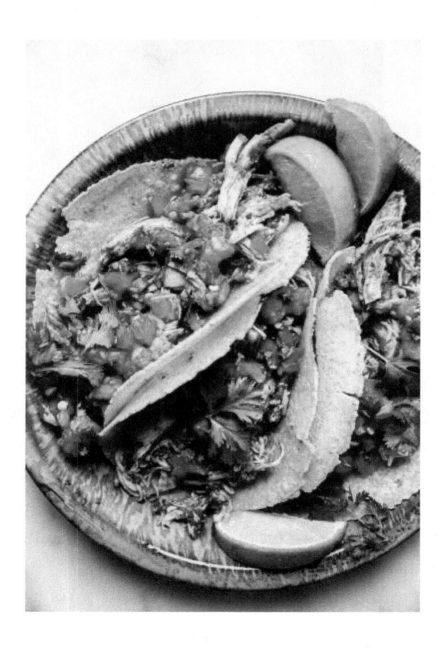

- <u>Crock-Pot Chicken Taco Meat</u>. Wait wait wait—taco night can be even easier? Yep! Meet our 3-ingredient Crock-Pot chicken taco meat recipe!
- <u>Mango Chutney Chicken Sheet Pan</u>. A jar of store-bought mango chutney is the secret to this ultra easy dinner.
- <u>Old Bay Shrimp and Sausage Sheet Pan Dinner</u>. Need we say more? Old Bay makes everything taste good—not that shrimp and sausage need any help.
- <u>Za'atar Chicken Sheet Pan Dinner</u>. We dressed up basic cauliflower and chicken with our latest favorite spice blend, za'atar.

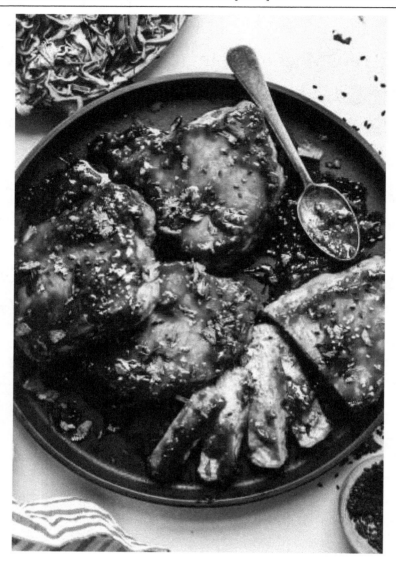

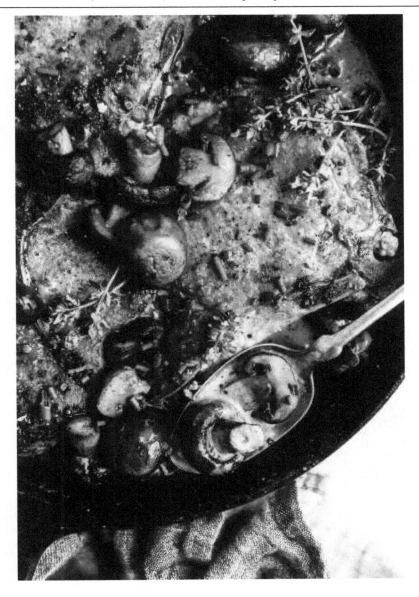

Pork & Sausage Make Everything Taste AMAZING.

- <u>Sausage, Kale and Potato Skillet Dinner</u>. An easy one-pan sausage, kale and potato skillet that pleases everyone, from cook to clean-up crew.

- <u>Hoisin Glazed Pork Chops</u>. Having a few punchy ingredients on-hand is a great way to make a simple dinner out of just a few ingredients. Hoisin sauce is one of our go-to super-ingredients for easy dinners—just slather it on some pork chops, and you're well on your way to dinnertime bliss.

- <u>Pork Chops with Mushroom Cream Sauce</u>. Speaking of pork chops, this version—with a super creamy mushroom sauce—is ready in just 30 minutes.

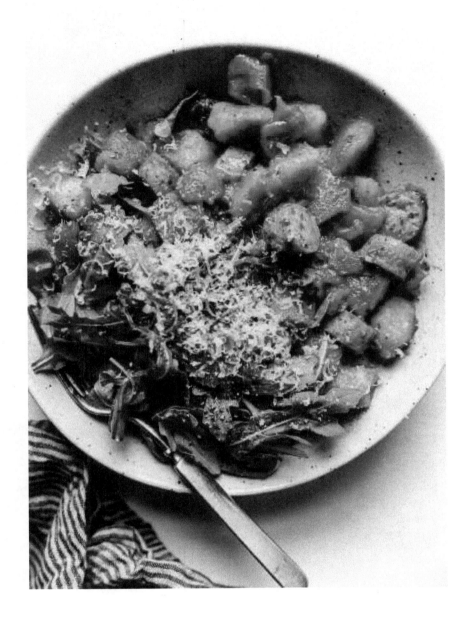

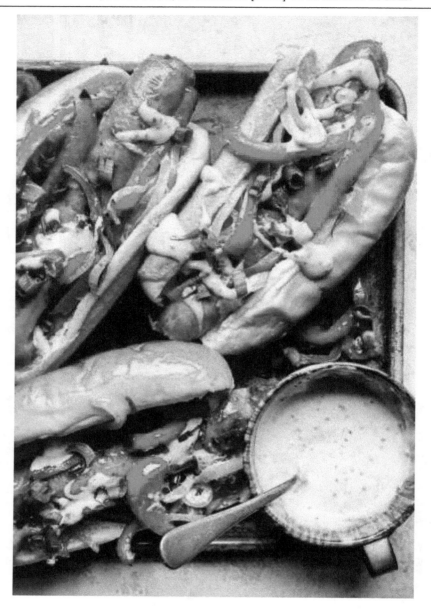

- Grilled Pork Tenderloin with Chimichurri. Grilling always makes for an easy dinner, right? It's so fast, and the cleanup is minimal. Sliced up this pork tenderloin and serve it with a bowl of chimichurri—you'll be hearing raves for days.

- Cauliflower Gnocchi with Bruschetta Sauce and Sausage. This hearty, low-carb supper that bursts with bright, bold flavors and comes together in under ten minutes. It just doesn't get easier or healthier than that!

- Sheet Pan Italian Sausage Heros with Honey Mustard. The brilliant thing about breaking out your sheet pan to make italian sausage sandwiches with peppers is that it makes it so easy to make Italian hoagies for a crowd! Gather the hungry masses and let the feeding begin.

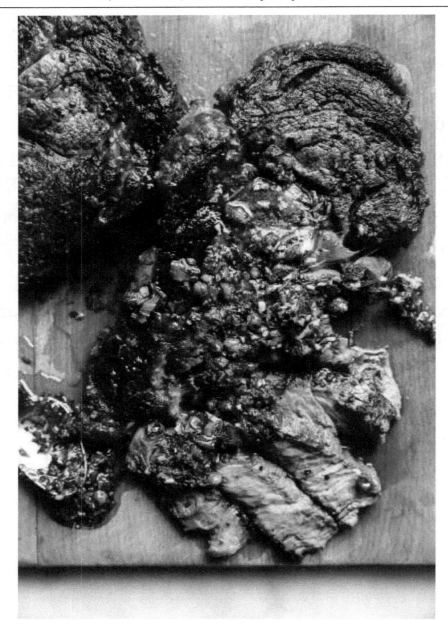

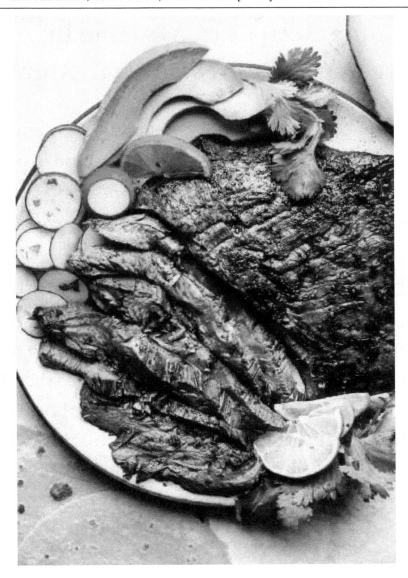

The Best Dinner Recipes of All Time Involve Steak — We Can All Agree on That, Right?

- Grilled Rib Eye Steak with Italian Salsa Verde. Easy? Check. Fast? Yup. Almost-no clean up? Uh, yeah, this recipe is perfect.
- Carne Asada. This easy carne asada recipe is as simple as can be — fire up the grill and you'll be feasting on juicy carne asada tacos in no time.
- Chimichurri Steak. For some reason, a perfectly grilled steak never fails to impress people. And it's really easy to do. Grab yourself about ten minutes, fire up the grill, and let's make a great steak!
- Grilled Five Spice Flank Steak. A Chinese five spice-hoisin marinade sinks into scored flank steak like nobody's business, and turns a simply grilled flank steak into a total flavor bomb.

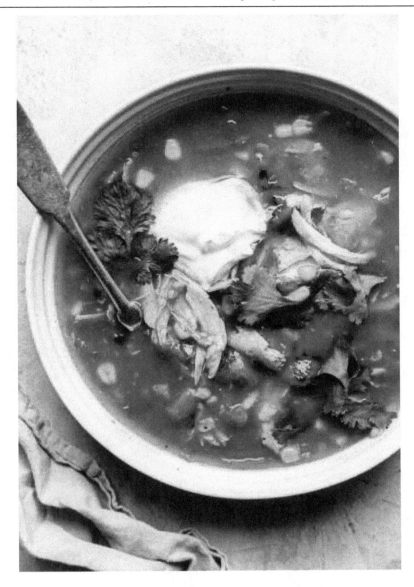

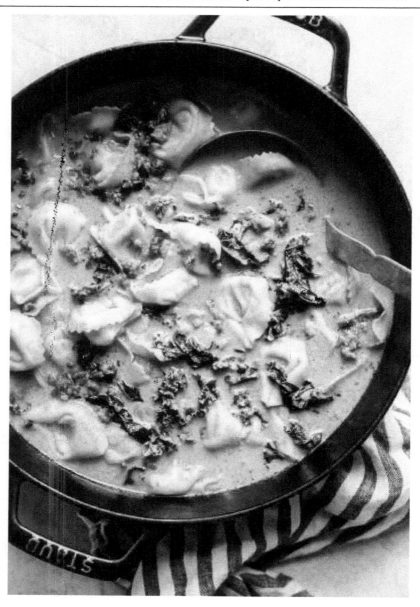

Soup!

- <u>5-Ingredient Chicken Tortilla Soup</u>. As simple and easy as it sounds. No, actually, it's even easier than that.
- <u>Taco Soup</u>. Like tacos, but soup! Seriously!
- <u>Tikka Masala Soup</u>. Your favorite Indian chicken recipe, soup-ified.
- <u>Tortellini Soup with Italian Sausage and Kale</u>. Can we just call this "The Soup"? A creamy tomato base is loaded with cheese tortellini and hearty sausage and basically this soup is just the greatest dinner ever.

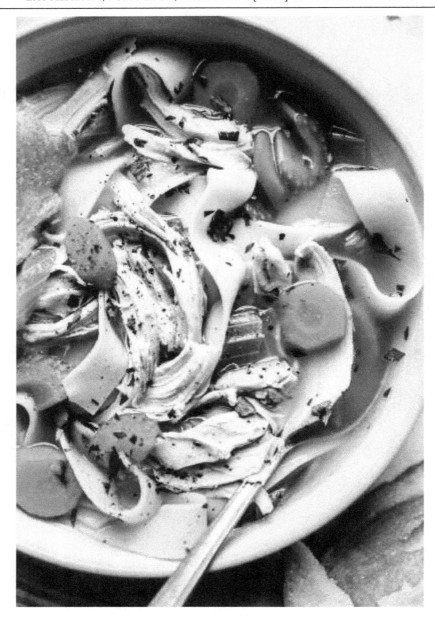

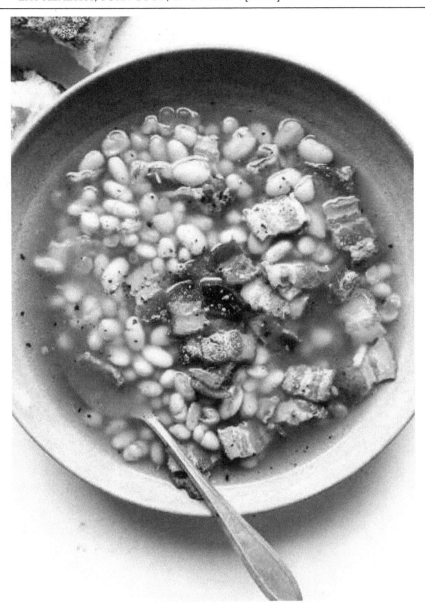

- <u>Quick and Easy Chicken Noodle Soup</u>. Just what it sounds like! Comfort in a pot.
- <u>Coconut Curry Ramen</u>. This restaurant-worthy creamy ramen is ready in about 15 minutes and is loaded with healthy veggies — in other words, it's a weeknight dream.
- <u>White Bean Soup with Bacon</u>. Creamy and deeply savory, it's hard to believe that this rich and hearty white bean soup with bacon is made from just five simple ingredients.

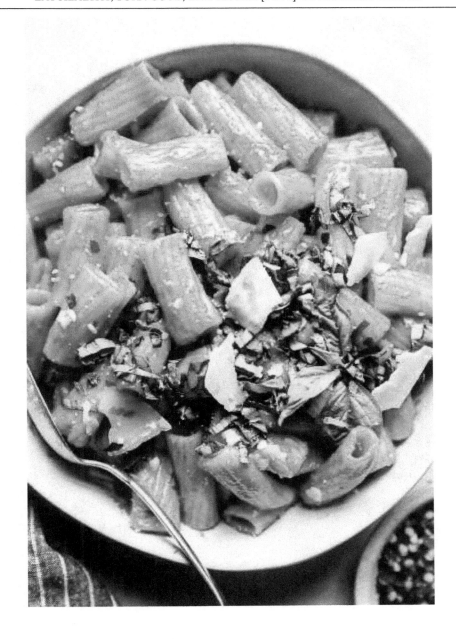

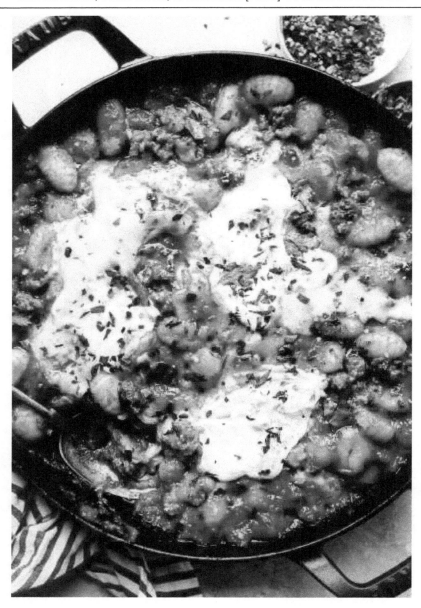

Oodles of Easy Noodle Recipes

- <u>Three-Ingredient Tomato Sauce</u>. Olive oil, salt, fresh tomatoes, and a little time are all it takes to create the most vibrant, fresh pasta sauce ever. Basic, easy, dinner perfection.

- <u>Creamy Roasted Red Pepper Pasta</u>. dinner doesn't get easier or more delicious than this creamy roasted red pepper rigatoni pasta. If you've got ten minutes and can open a jar, you can make this tonight.

- <u>4-Ingredient Stovetop Macaroni and Cheese</u>. Easy homemade mac and cheese is just ten minutes (and four ingredients!) away. So what are you waiting for?

- <u>Baked Gnocchi</u>. A skillet full of melty, bubbly, carb-y comfort is just what the dreary, drizzly weeknights ahead need to perk them up.

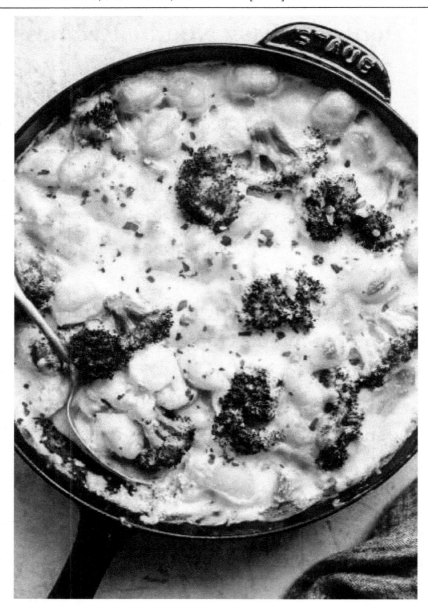

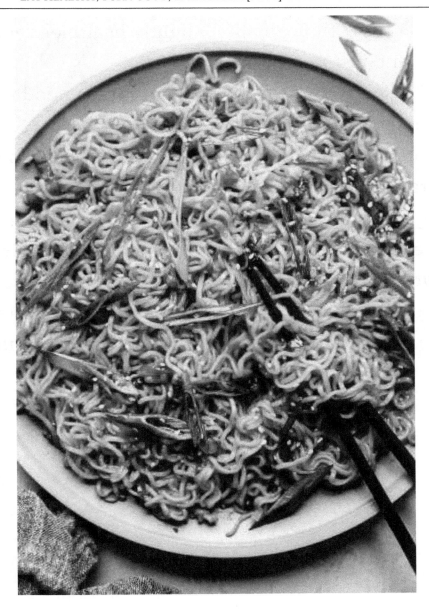

- Baked Gnocchi with Broccoli. A slightly healthier version, but just as cheesy, and just as easy.
- Sesame Garlic Ramen Noodles. Instant ramen noodles make this super simple dinner even faster.
- Brown Butter Sage Cauliflower Gnocchi. TJ's cauliflower gnocchi have literally never tasted so good.
- Easy Bolognese. Hearty and comforting, this meaty, easy bolognese sauce recipe takes less time to make than it does to disappear into hungry tummies.
- Shrimp Scampi. Buttery, garlicky, shrimp-y, and pasta-y (if you want it to be). Got 15 minutes? Great. Let's make shrimp scampi!

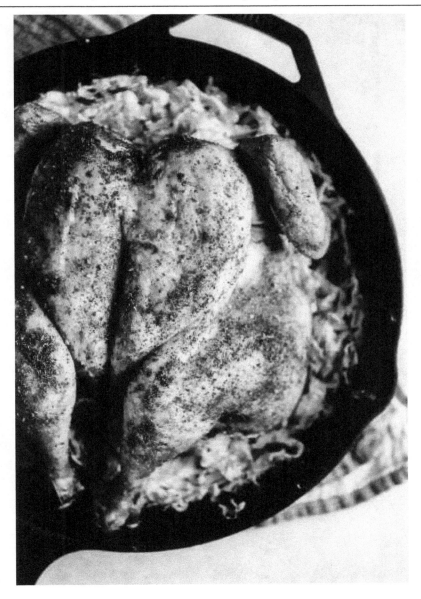

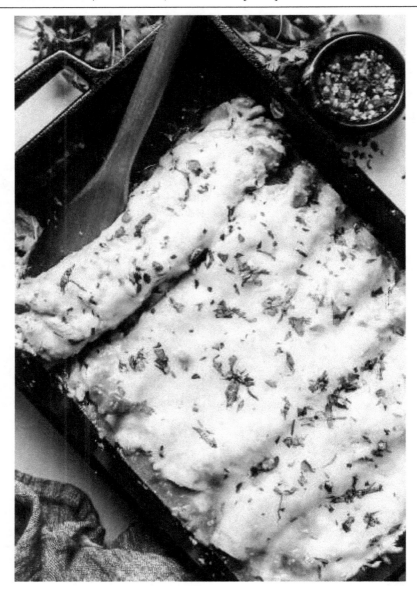

Dinner Ideas

Easy Harissa Chicken. Easy, quick harissa chicken—made with a jar of roasted red peppers, plenty of garlic, and smoked paprika—is a lot more exciting than any chicken recipe has any right to be.

- Cilantro-Lime Chicken Thighs. A quick marinade of lime, garlic, bright cilantro, and a touch of honey transforms boneless, skinless chicken thighs into just the juicy, tender surge of sunshine that you crave.

- Skillet Roasted Chicken with Cabbage. Easy delicious dinners win every time in our book. This one-pan whole roasted chicken falls into that easy category.

- Green Chicken Enchiladas. Our easy green chicken enchilada recipe is weeknight ready and all but guaranteed to please everyone from starving spouses to picky toddlers.

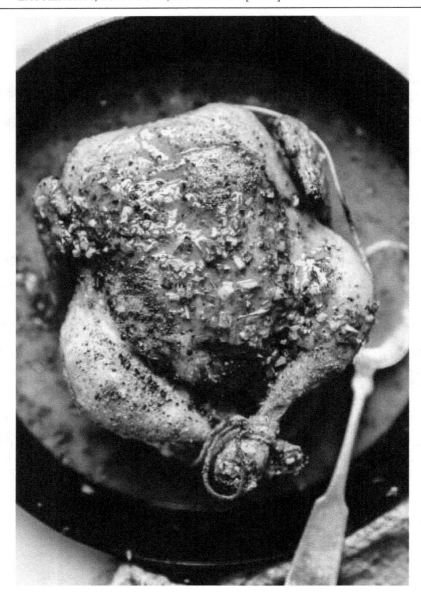

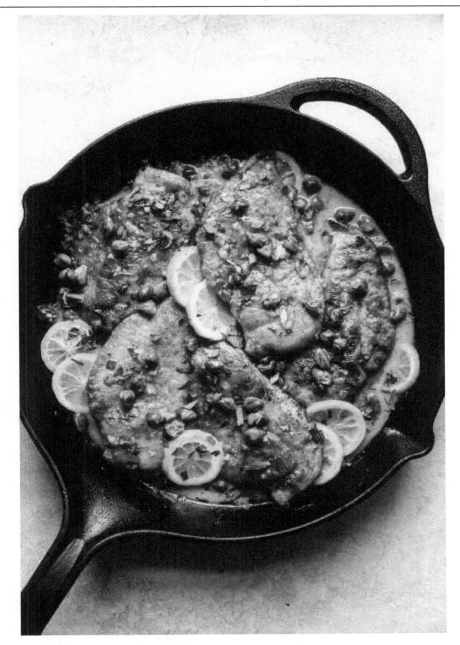

- <u>Perfect Roast Chicken with Lemon Herb Pan Sauce</u>. The original easy dinner—roast chicken. No sweat, no stress and GREAT leftovers. What's not to love?
- <u>Whole Roast Chicken with Carrots</u>. Same as above but with carrots! Um, yum.
- <u>Greek Chicken Freezer Meal</u>. Freezer meals are *future* easy meals, and this one is a real winner of a chicken dinner.

- <u>Freezer Chicken Fajitas</u>. Fajitas are easy anytime, but especially if you did most of the work a few months ago. Freezer meals FTW!
- <u>Chicken Piccata</u>. We just love recipes like this—not shortcuts required, because the classic recipe happens to be naturally fast and easy.

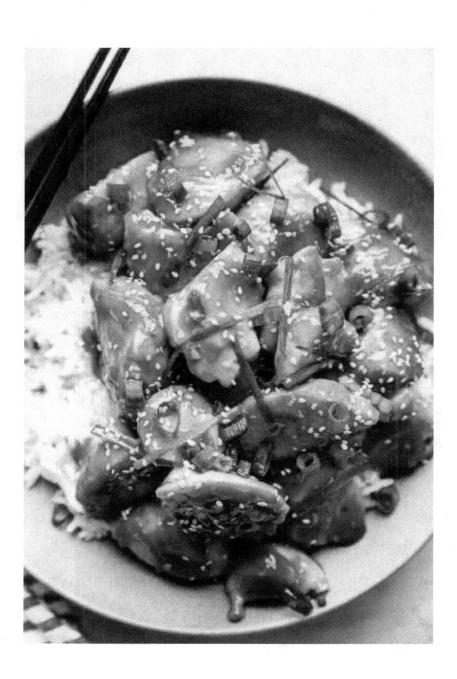

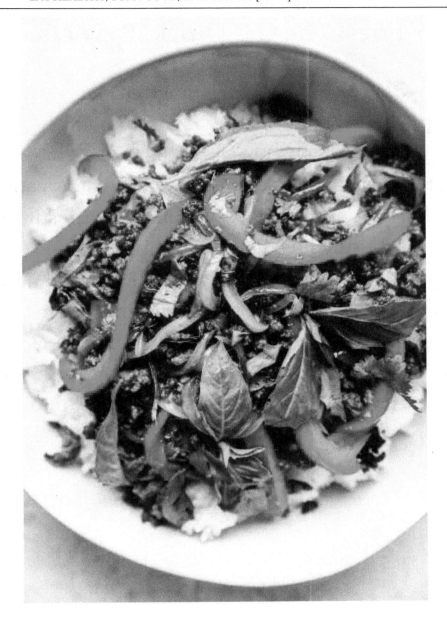

Stir-Fries: The OG Quick, Easy Dinner

- <u>Easy Orange Chicken</u>. Our easy orange chicken recipe puts a healthy spin on the sweet-savory favorite.

- <u>Kung Pao Chicken</u>. Step away from the takeout menu. Step towards the stove and make this easy chicken instead!

- <u>Thai Basil Beef</u>. A speedy, savory Thai beef basil stir fry that's just a bit spicy and really hits the spot.

- <u>Crispy Chicken Stir Fry</u>. Cornstarch and high heat mean super-crispy chicken every time. Toss in some green beans, and you've got an easy, healthy dinner in about 10 minutes.

- <u>Gingery Ground Beef (Soboro Donburi)</u>. Five ingredients, a few minutes and a hot skillet, and you'll be digging into a delicious soboro donburi.

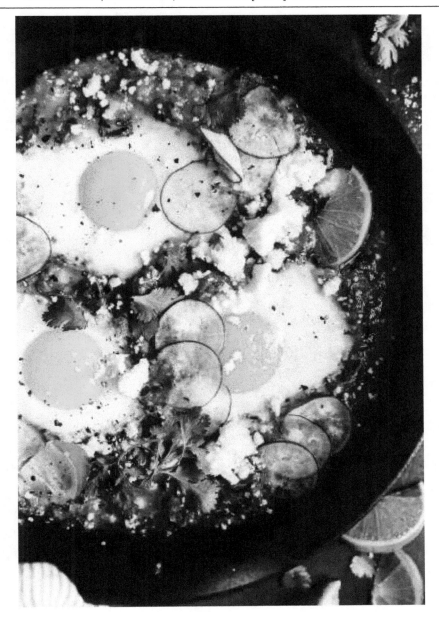

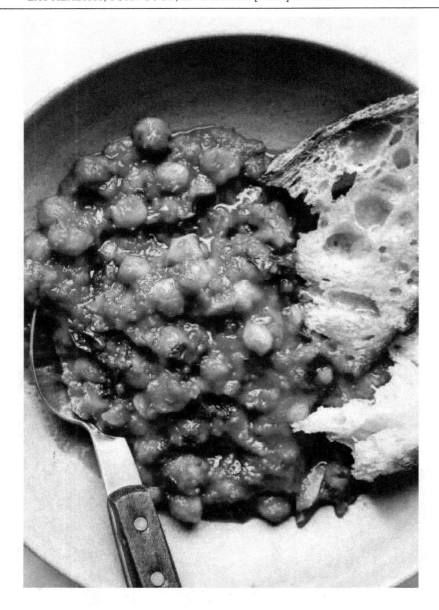

Easy, Fast Vegetarian Dinner Ideas

- <u>Salsa Verde Baked Eggs</u>. A jar of salsa verde makes this elegant egg dish incredibly speedy. Yeah, it sounds brunchy, but trust us—try it for dinner!

- <u>Braised Chickpeas with Chard</u>. Rich, filling and healthy, this dinner is as fast and delicious as any we could imagine. Easy on the budget, too!

- <u>Portobello Mushroom Fajitas</u>. Just as good as their chicken or steak-filled counterparts, and just as fast, too.

- <u>Huevos Rancheros</u>. Runny, fried eggs over a bed of seasoned beans, atop a layer of warm corn tortillas, add a few condiments and voila—breakfast for dinner takes on a whole new meaning.

- <u>Soft-Scrambled Eggs</u>. Don't knock it—scrambled eggs make a perfect dinner in our book. Add a little salad if you want to round it out, and dinner will still be ready in about 10 minutes.

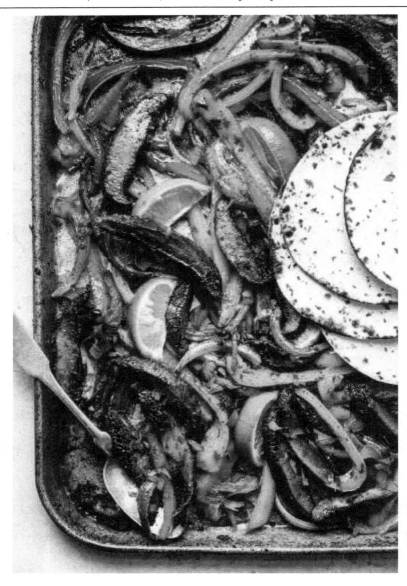

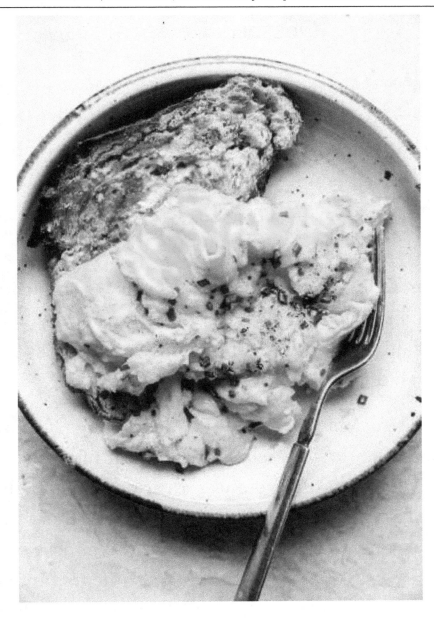

Desserts Recipes

A piece of what makes the Mediterranean diet so mainstream is the manner by which adaptable it is. You don't need to tally carbs or do any math to follow it. However long you're eating new foods grown from the ground with each supper, and picking entire grains over refined flours, you can enjoy different things.

Red meat is alright every so often, and you can eat fish and chicken a couple of times each week. The diet is normally high in plant-based protein from chickpeas, beans, and entire grains and you'll get a ton of your energy from sound fats and complex sugars that require a significant stretch of time to process.

Studies show this diet can do some incredible things for your wellbeing. That incorporates lower cholesterol, diminished danger for cardiovascular illness, and weight reduction. Obviously, there's no assurance you'll get these advantages, and there are alternate approaches to accomplish your wellbeing and wellness objectives other than restricting your diet to these nourishments. Indeed, the best wellbeing and wellness plan is the one that is nicely obliged the food sources you like to eat and the exercises you most appreciate.

Exacting diets can devour your day. What's more, from various perspectives, they can be similarly pretty much as undesirable as thoughtlessly or enthusiastically eating. All things considered, making little, insightful decisions for the duration of the day can improve your wellbeing without overwhelming your musings. Furthermore, that is the thing that this book is here for. We can help you structure an arrangement that leaves space for you to carry on with your life.

With this book, you get an individual wellbeing mentor who endeavors to help you make SMART objectives (that is Specific, Measurable, Attainable, Realistic and Time-situated) so you can remain persuaded all through the cycle. What's more, our caring local area gives you the help you need to remain on target. In the event that the correct diet for you incorporates some sugar – that is OK! We can represent that together. The Mediterranean diet is about balance, which implies dessert is not really impossible. Fixings like new organic product, olive oil, and yogurt are staples with regards to desserts, bringing about desserts that are light, new, and brimming with flavor. Like such a large amount of Mediterranean cooking, desserts are infrequently muddled, frequently meeting up in one bowl with only a couple fixings. Here are 10 of delicious and healthy Mediterranean dessert plans.

1. Blood Orange Olive Oil Cake

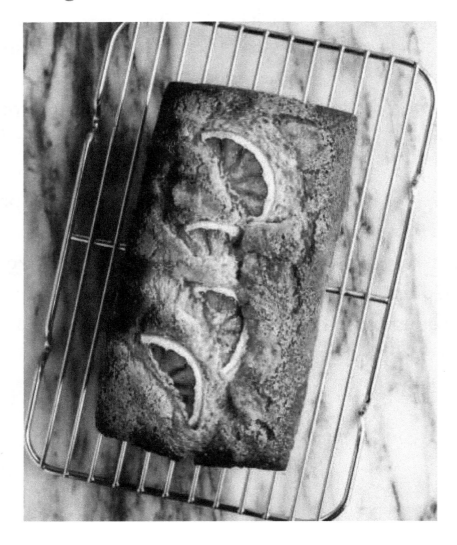

This cake is an ensemble of straightforward tastes additional virgin olive oil contributes a fruity nose, while a controlled measure of sugar clears a path for the pith of the blood orange, with its perplexing pleasantness and fragrant, clashing zing coming through in each nibble.

On the off chance that blood oranges aren't accessible, Cara or normal oranges make a pleasant substitute, since you'll be eating the whole natural product zing and all attempt to source natural citrus whenever the situation allows.

INGREDIENTS

- Cooking splash or extra-virgin olive oil
- 1 medium blood orange
- 1/4 cups generally useful flour
- 1/2 cup medium-crush cornmeal
- 2 teaspoons preparing powder
- 1/4 teaspoon preparing pop
- 1/4 teaspoon fine salt
- 2/3 cup in addition to 2 tablespoons granulated sugar, separated
- 1/2 cup entire milk plain yogurt
- 3 huge eggs
- 1/2 cup extra-virgin olive oil
- 4 paper-slim half-moon-formed blood orange cuts (discretionary)

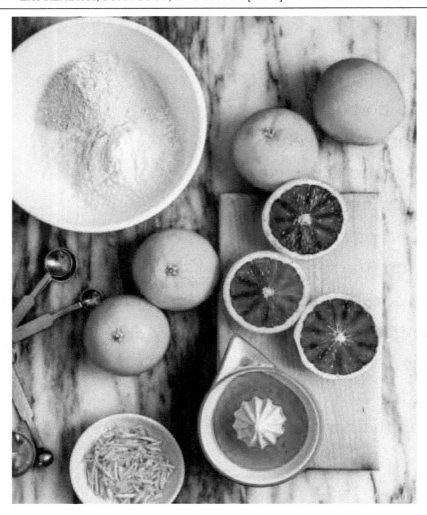

INSTRUCTIONS

- Orchestrate a rack in the broiler and warmth to 350°F. Oil a 9-by 5-inch portion skillet with cooking splash or oil; put in a safe spot.

- Utilizing a vegetable peeler, eliminate the zing from the orange. Cut the zing into slender strips and put in a safe spot. Juice the orange and put aside 1/4 cup (save the leftover juice for utilization).

- Whisk the flour, cornmeal, heating powder, preparing pop, and salt together in a medium bowl; put in a safe spot.

- Whisk 2/3 cup of the sugar and the 1/4 cup blood orange squeeze together in enormous bowl. Each in turn, speeds in the yogurt, eggs, and olive oil. Whisk the flour combination into the wet ingredients, giving the blend 20 great turns with the speed until just joined. Overlap in the zing strips.

- Move the hitter into the readied skillet. Top with the blood orange cuts and staying 2 tablespoons sugar. Heat until the top is springy and brilliant earthy colored, and a wooden stick embedded in the middle comes out with only a couple morsels joined, 50 to an hour.

Allow the cake to cool in the dish on a wire rack for 20 minutes. Cautiously unmold the cake, flip it back to be straight up, and get back to the rack to cool totally.

Balsamic Berries with Honey Yogurt

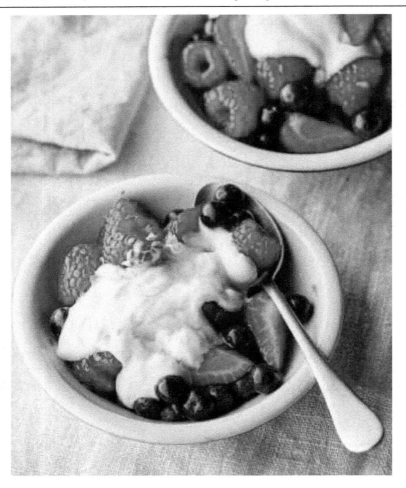

It might appear to be nonsensical to throw berries in vinegar for dessert; however in the event that you've at any point attempted this mix, you realize how well it works. Balsamic vinegar, while tart, has a characteristic pleasantness to it. At the point when showered over strawberries, blueberries, and raspberries, it draws a portion of the normal squeezes and sugars out of the natural product to make profoundly seasoned syrup for them to swim in. Much the same as that, the berries are an ideal method to cover off a dinner, however completing them with a touch of nectar improved yogurt certainly doesn't do any harm. Select entire milk plain Greek yogurt for the most velvety lavishness.

INGREDIENTS

- 8 ounces strawberries, hulled and split, or quartered if extremely enormous (around 1/2 cups)
- 1 cup blueberries
- 1 cup raspberries
- 1 tablespoon balsamic vinegar
- 2/3 cup entire milk plain Greek yogurt

2 teaspoons nectar

INSTRUCTIONS

Throw the strawberries, blueberries, and raspberries with the balsamic vinegar in a huge bowl. Let it sit for 10 minutes. Mix the yogurt and nectar together in a little bowl. Split the berries between serving bowls or glasses and top each with a spot of nectar yogurt.

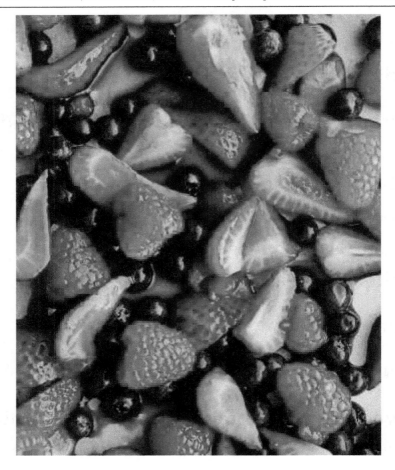

Sticky Gluten-Free Lemon Cake

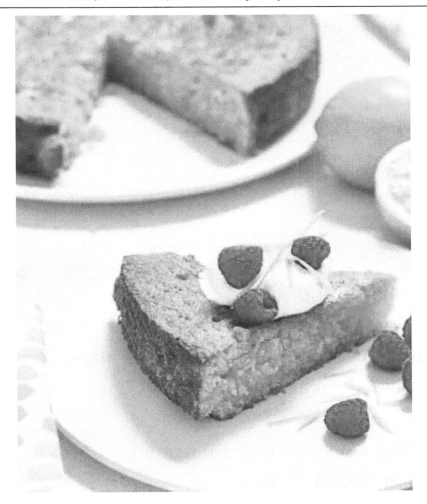

Warm cake and warm syrup are the things that make this lemony cake so sodden and tasty. Ensure you jab a lot of openings in the cake so the syrup gets an opportunity to douse into each and every nibble of cake as it cools. I realize it'll be difficult to be persistent, however stand by until the cake cools totally with the goal that all the flavors truly get an opportunity to merge and you'll be remunerated. This cake is heated in a spring structure search for gold evacuation for cutting (when the syrup goes on, it's difficult to eliminate from the container in one piece). You can positively make it in a normal cake dish, yet it will presumably be ideal to cut and teach it a thing or two out of the container. This cake is incredible all alone, yet stunningly better with a touch of frothy whipped cream on top!

INGREDIENTS

For the cake:

- 2 cups almond flour
- 3/4 cup polenta
- 1/2 teaspoons heating powder
- 1/4 teaspoon salt
- 14 tablespoons (7 ounces) unsalted margarine, at room temperature, in addition to additional for the skillet
- 1 cup granulated sugar
- 3 enormous eggs
- Finely ground zing of 2 medium lemons
- 1/2 teaspoon vanilla concentrate

For the syrup and serving:

- 1/2 cup powdered sugar
- 3 tablespoons newly crushed lemon juice
- Whipped cream, for serving (discretionary)

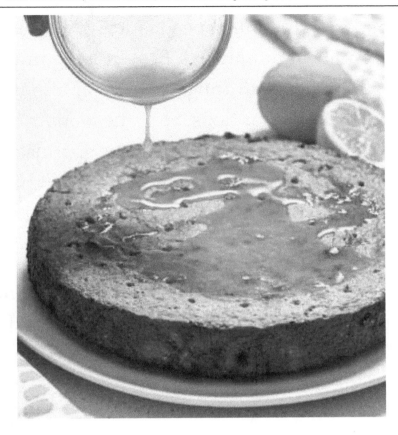

INSTRUCTIONS

For cake:

- Organize a rack in the stove and warmth to 350°F. Line the lower part of a 9-inch spring form skillet with material paper. Coat the paper and sides of the container with margarine; put in a safe spot.
- Spot the almond flour, polenta, heating powder, and salt in a medium bowl and race to consolidate; put in a safe spot.
- Spot the margarine and sugar in the bowl of a stand blender fitted with the oar connection. (Then again, utilize an electric hand blender and huge bowl.) Beat on medium speed until helped in shading, around 3 minutes.

- With the blender on medium speed, add 1/3 of the almond flour combination and beat until fused. Beat in 1 egg until consolidated. Keep beating in and substituting the leftover almond flour blend and eggs in 2 additional options. Stop the blender and scratch down the sides of the bowl with an elastic spatula.
- Add the lemon zing and vanilla concentrate and beat until just consolidated. Move the hitter to the container and spread into an even layer.

Heat until the edges of the cake has started to pull away from the sides of the skillet, around 40 minutes. Spot the skillet on a wire rack and make the syrup.

For the syrup:

- Spot the powdered sugar and lemon juice in a little pot over low warmth and cook, mixing periodically, until the powdered sugar is totally broken up and the syrup is warm. Eliminate from the warmth.
- Utilizing a toothpick, punch holes everywhere on the cake, dispersing the openings around 1-inch separated. Gradually shower the warm syrup uniformly over the cake. Allow the cake to cool totally, around 1/2 hours. Eliminate the sides of the skillet, cut into wedges, and present with whipped cream whenever wanted.

2. Honeyed Phyllo Stacks with Pistachios, Spiced Fruit & Yogurt

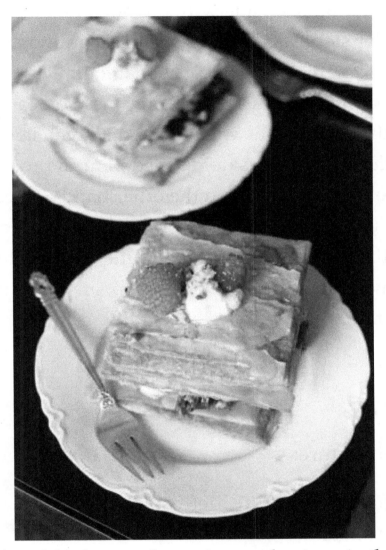

- One of the old adages of evening gatherings is this: Do not cause a recipe interestingly when you to have visitors coming over. However, a few recipes are an exemption, similar to this one, which I tried interestingly on a full table of visitors. They cherished its layers of shatteringly fresh phyllo, the light whirls of yogurt, and the filling of hacked raisins, nectar, and pistachios rather like a lighter, deconstructed baklava.

- Here's something intriguing about phyllo, as well: I gained from one of our perusers that phyllo batter is really vegetarian it's made with oil, not spread. This adaptable cooler staple is additionally an accommodating part for amassing liked up desserts that look wonderful yet are really a snap to make, similar to this one. You can make little cakes with the batter, as we do here and even layer them with delicate cheddar, safeguarded natural product, and sweet-smelling nectar. Or on the other hand you can proceed to make a veggie lover dessert by avoiding the dairy yogurt and utilizing coconut yogurt all things considered, and subbing agave, earthy colored rice syrup, or sorghum syrup for the nectar.

INGREDIENTS

For the phyllo mixture:

- 6 sheets phyllo mixture, defrosted
- 1/4 cup sugar
- 1/4 teaspoon ground cinnamon
- 1/4 cup extra-virgin olive oil
- For the pistachio and organic product blend:
- Zing and juice of 1 orange (around 1/4 cup juice)
- 2 tablespoons sugar
- 2 tablespoons nectar
- 1/2 cup dried brilliant raisins, generally cleaved
- 1 cup cooked unsalted pistachio nuts, generally cleaved

- 1/2 cup pitted dates, generally cleaved
- 1/2 teaspoon ground cardamom
- **For yogurt:**
- 1 cup entire milk Greek yogurt
- 1 tablespoon confectioners' sugar
- Zing of 1 lemon
- **For serving:**
- 1/2 cup pomegranate arils
- 1/4 cup pistachios, cleaved
- Nectar, warmed
- Raspberries or strawberries to decorate, discretionary
-

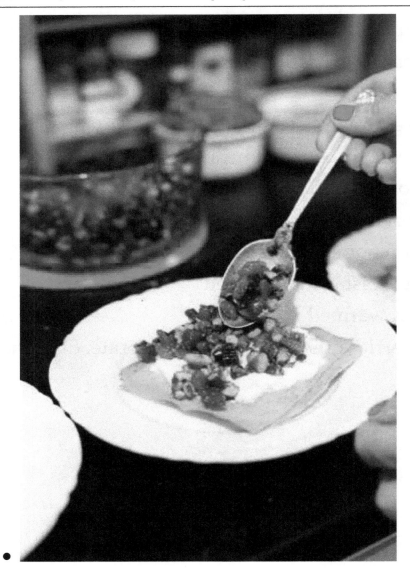

INSTRUCTIONS

To set up the phyllo squares:

Preheat the broiler to 400°F and fix an enormous preparing sheet with material.

- Stack the phyllo sheets on the ledge and cover freely with a scarcely soggy towel. Join the sugar and cinnamon in a little bowl. Put the oil in another little bowl. Eliminate a sheet of phyllo and spot it on the readied preparing sheet. Utilizing a cake brush, gently cover the phyllo mixture with the olive oil and sprinkle softly with the cinnamon sugar. Top with another sheet of phyllo, oil, and cinnamon sugar. Rehash with the entirety of the sheets, yet when you get to the top layer, brushes it gently with oil. Use kitchen shears to clip the layered mixture into 12 squares or square shapes of equivalent size.

- Heat the phyllo batter for 7 to 8 minutes or until it is brilliant earthy colored and fresh. Allow it to cool totally. The readied phyllo squares can be put away in a water/air proof holder at room temperature for as long as 3 days.

- **For pistachio and fruit mix:**
- In a little pot, heat the orange zing and orange squeeze, sugar, and nectar until the juice boils and the nectar breaks down. Mix in the brilliant raisins and put the dish in a safe spot.

Blend the pistachios in with the dates. Mix in the cardamom. Mix the spiced pistachios and dates into the container with the syrup and raisins. Put aside the pistachio and organic product blend to marinate for in any event 30 minutes. This combination can be made as long as 5 days early and put away in the fridge.

For yogurt:
Altogether blend the yogurt in with the confectioners' sugar and lemon zing. The yogurt combination can be refrigerated for as long as 5 days, all around covered.

For dessert:
- Smear around 1 tablespoon of yogurt on a phyllo cake square. Spot on an individual dessert plate. Top with a liberal spoonful of

the organic product combination, at that point another phyllo square. Rehash, and top with a last cake square and a little dab of yogurt. Sprinkle the stack and the dish around it with pomegranate arils and pistachios; at that point shower delicately with warmed nectar. Rehash, making 4 phyllo square stacks, and serve right away. Enhancement whenever wanted with occasional organic product like raspberries or strawberries.

Fig and pistachio cake

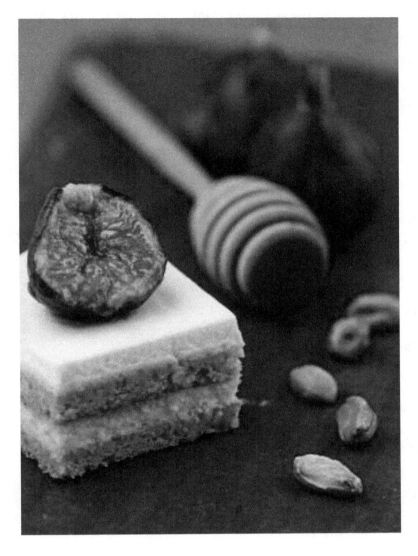

You don't have to roast them; they are a perfectly fine accompaniment on their own. But the thought of honey-scented figs just upped the autumn factor for me. They are also really good by themselves, if you don't have time to make a cake. Pistachios ready for pulverizing. The cake is essentially a Genoese, made nutty with pistachios and moistened with sugar syrup. I found the mascarpone cream had a weight and tang that contrasted nicely with the light sponge cake, more so than just a basic whipped cream filling. I also didn't want to make the cake too sweet, as the figs-and-honey was already providing plenty of sweetness.

Ingredients

For pistachio cake

- 40 g pistachios
- 75 g powdered sugar
- 40 g blanched almonds
- 40 g egg yolks
- 60 g eggs
- 115 g egg whites
- 2 g cream of tartar
- 50 g + 1/2 cup sugar
- 60 g all-purpose flour

For mascarpone frosting

- 1 cup heavy cream
- 8 oz. mascarpone cheese
- 1/2 cup powdered sugar

For roasted figs

- About 12 ripe figs
- 1 tablespoon unsalted butter
- 2 tablespoons honey

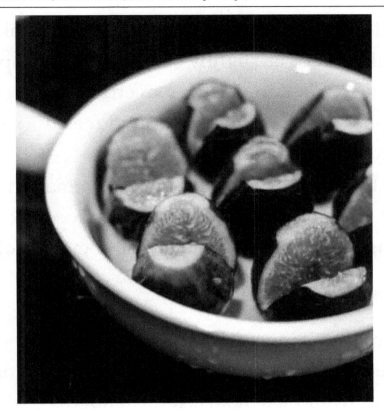

Instructions

For the cake:

- Preheat oven to 425 degrees F. Grease two 8x8 pans, line with parchment paper, and grease parchment paper.
- Combine pistachios, powdered sugar, and almonds in a food processor. Process until nuts are finely ground.
- Pour nut mixture into a large mixing bowl. Add in eggs and egg yolks and stir until combined.
- Combine egg whites, cream of tartar, and 2 tablespoons of the 50 g of sugar in bowl of a stand mixer. Whip until soft peaks form. Add remaining sugar and whisk until stiff peaks.
- Sift the flour over the nut mixture and stir to combine. Add in the egg whites and carefully fold in.

- Divide the batter between the two pans. Bake for 8-10 minutes until the tops are lightly colored and the top just springs back to the touch. Remove from oven and place on wire racks. Run an offset spatula or knife around the edges to loosen the cake from the pans. Let cool.
- For the sugar syrup: Combine the remaining 1/2 cup sugar and 1/2 cup water in a medium saucepan on the stove and bring to a boil, stirring to let the sugar dissolve. Let cool.

For mascarpone frosting:

- Combine all ingredients in bowl of a stand mixer. Whisk together until soft peaks form. Add more confectioner's sugar if you would like it sweeter. Do not over whisk or the mixture will curdle.
- To assemble the cake: Trim off the edges of each square of edge to even them off. Place one layer of cake on a plate. Brush a little of sugar syrup over the cake layer. Spread a layer of frosting evenly on top. Place second layer of cake on frosting and brush sugar syrup over it. Spread a layer of frosting evenly on top.
- Refrigerate cake for about an hour or so to let frosting set. When you are ready to serve the cake, you can take it out and trim the sides so they look nice and even.

For the figs:

- Preheat oven to 425 degrees F. Wash figs and slice them in half. Arrange in an ovenproof baking dish just large enough to fit them.

- Combine butter and honey in a small saucepan and cook over medium heat on the stove until butter is melted. Pour over the figs.
- Place figs in oven and bake for about 13-15 minutes, until the sauce is bubbling. Remove figs and let cool on wire rack for a few minutes before serving.

Vegan Chocolate Chip Cookies

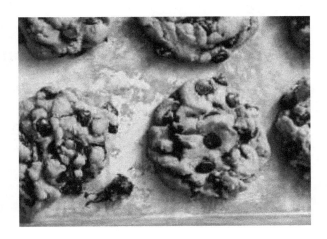

Ingredients:

- 2 cup all-purpose flour
- 1 tsp. baking soda
- 1/2 tsp. kosher salt
- 1/2 cup dark brown sugar
- 1/2 cup granulated sugar
- 1/2 cup canola oil
- 1/4 cup water
- 2 tsp. pure vanilla extract
- 1 cup bittersweet chocolate chips

1 cup semisweet chocolate chips

Instructions

- In a bowl, mix salt, baking soda, and flour. Toss with chocolate. In another bowl, break up brown sugar, making sure there are no lumps. Add granulated sugar, oil, water, and vanilla and whisk to combine. Add flour mixture and mix until just completely mixed (there should be no streaks of flour). Put two cookie sheets with parchment paper. Spoon out 2-inch mounds of dough, spacing 2 inches apart. Freeze 30 minutes.

Preheat oven to 375°F. Bake cookies, rotating position of pans after 6 minutes until edges are golden brown, 9 to 12 minutes total. Let cool.

Cinnamon Walnut Apple Cake Baked with Olive Oil

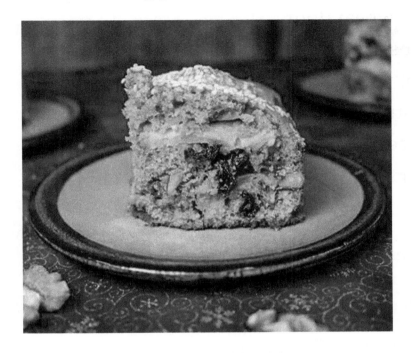

We utilize olive oil for everything, including heating desserts (Mediterranean Diet recipes traditionally utilize olive oil for preparing). This cinnamon pecan apple cake has been heated for exceptional events in my family for ages. Despite the fact that we have natural product for dessert on most evenings, we will make this as a treat when we are celebrating. Olive oil makes for smooth and clammy prepared merchandise and I would energetically suggest it for the vast majority of your heating needs. One tip is to attempt to get a rich or fruity enhanced olive oil when you are heating. Eat this cake with evening tea or espresso or after a quick bite.

Ingredients

- 4 eggs
- 1 cup earthy colored sugar (in addition to 2 Tablespoons for apples)
- 1 cup additional virgin olive oil

- 1 cup milk
- 2 1/2 cups wheat flour
- 2 teaspoons preparing powder
- 1 teaspoon vanilla concentrate
- 4 apples, stripped, split, cored, and daintily cut
- 1/2 cup pecans, cleaved
- 1/2 cup raisins
- 1/2 teaspoons ground cinnamon

3 tablespoons sesame seeds

Instructions

- Preheat stove to 375 degrees.
- Beat eggs and sugar with a hand blender for 10 minutes. Add olive oil and beat for an extra 3 minutes.
- Add milk, wheat flour, preparing powder and vanilla. Beat for 2 minutes.
- Brush a 9" cake container with olive oil. Add a large portion of the hitter to the skillet.
- In a bowl, blend apples, 2 tablespoons of earthy colored sugar, pecans, raisins and cinnamon. Pour apple combination on top of hitter in cake skillet.
- Add remaining hitter to container and sprinkle with sesame seeds.
- Heat for 45-50 minutes until embedded blade confesses all.

3. Vanilla Cake Bites

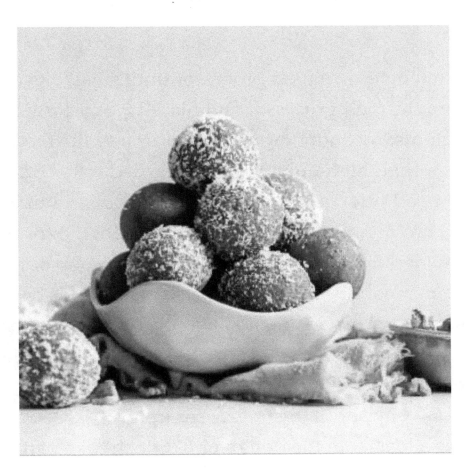

Ingredients:

- 1 1/4 cups Medjool dates

- 1 1/4 cups raw walnuts

- 1 cup almond flour

- 1/3 cup coconut flour

- Pinch sea salt

- Two teaspoon vanilla extract

Finely shredded unsweetened coconut *(optional)*

Intructions

- Pulse pitted dates in a food processor until small bits remain. Take it out from the food processor and placed it apart. Add the almond flour, walnuts, coconut flour, and sea salt into the food processor. Blend till a semi-high-quality meal is carried out. Add dates returned in addition to the vanilla extract. Pulse until loose dough form. Be careful not to over-blend. You're looking for pliable dough, not a purée. Using a cookie scooper, scoop out 2-Tablespoon amounts and roll into balls with hands or release lever on the scoop and place directly on a parchment-lined baking sheet. Repeat until all dough is used up. Roll in finely shredded coconut, or leave it as is. Store in refrigerator or freezer. Keep in the fridge for up to 6-7 days or in the freezer for up to 3-4 weeks. You can also make a loaf from the dough or 6×6-inch cake pan and slice it into bars.

GREEK YOGURT CHOCOLATE MOUSSE

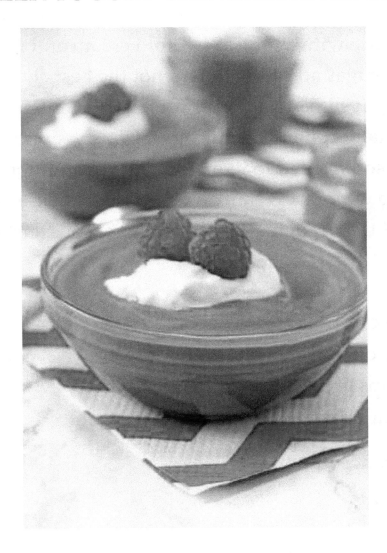

Chocolate Mousse must be a definitive in enticing dessert recipes. Rich and chocolaty there is something just so fulfilling about it. In any case, given that it's made with a tone of twofold cream and frequently a hill of refined white sugar additionally, it's not the best choice out there so I set about making it somewhat better for us. Conventional chocolate mousse additionally contains crude eggs. I wasn't excited about offering this to the child so I needed to likewise make a rendition that was sans egg. Without the whipped cream and eggs this mousse will not interpretation of that trademark light and vaporous surface.

INGREDIENTS

- 180ml/3/4 cup milk
- 100g/3 1/2 oz dull chocolate
- 500ml/2 cups greek yogurt
- 1 tbsp nectar or maple syrup

1/2 tsp vanilla concentrate

INSTRUCTIONS

- Empty the milk into a pot and add the chocolate, either ground or finely cleaved or shaved. Tenderly warmth the milk until the chocolate softens, being mindful so as not to allow it to boil. When the chocolate and milk have completely joined, add the nectar and vanilla concentrate and blend well.
- Spoon the greek yogurt into a huge bowl and pour the chocolate blend on top. Combine as one well prior to moving to singular dishes, ramekins or glasses.
- Chill in the ice chest for 2 hours. Present with a little spoonful of greek yogurt and some new raspberries.

- The chocolate mousse will keep in the cooler for 2 days.

Peanut Butter Protein Balls

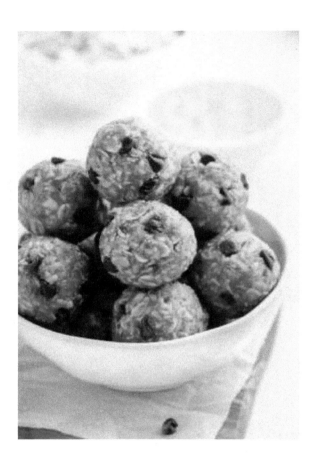

Ingredients

- 1 cup large Medjool dates pitted

- 2-4 tablespoons water

- 1 cup peanut flour

- 3/4 cup oats

- 1/2 cup roasted peanuts

- 1/4 cup natural peanut butter

- 2 tablespoons flax seeds ground into meal

- pinch of salt

- 1/4 cup chocolate chips optional

Instructions

Put the pitted dates in about 2 cups of water for 25- 30 minutes. Drain, reserving the water. In a food processor combination dates with 2-four tablespoons of water, slowly adding water as wanted and scraping down the edges frequently till a paste has formed. Add peanut butter, peanuts, salt, flax seeds, peanut flour, and oats and blend together into a thick dough. Round out about 2 tbsp. of dough into balls and place on a parchment-lined baking sheet. Refrigerate for 1 hour until firm. Store in an airtight container in refrigerator up to 5 days or in the freezer for 1 month.

The 15-Day Men's Health Book of 15-Minute Workouts

The Time-Saving Program to Raise a Leaner, Stronger, More Muscular You

Anphora Cooper

Table of Contents

Introduction

The 15-minute workout is a revolutionary idea. Most of us have been taught that a good workout takes 45 to 60 minutes, three or four times a week. But the benefits we get from the time spent exercising last only as long as we can push ourselves—and sometimes even less than that. Even those who exercise six days a week for 50 minutes each time rarely lose weight, build muscle or gain strength to any significant degree because their bodies adapt quickly to the demands they are placing on them. That's why I've developed this 15-minute program so you can get stronger, leaner and healthier without having to spend hours at the gym. You'll get leaner, stronger and better at burning off body fat—and you'll do it in less time than it takes to watch an hour-long TV series.

The 15-minute workout is based on simple exercise science. Researchers have known for decades that our bodies adapt quickly to the demands we place on them through exercise. When that happens, we stop getting as much benefit from the workouts we're doing. It's a concept called overtraining or spiking cortisol levels: The stress of regular workouts increases your cortisol levels, which makes you tired when you should be energized. Over time, you will stop seeing progress because your muscles will begin to stop responding to the training. The only way to overcome this adaptation is to keep increasing the intensity of your workouts—and that can spell trouble for your body.

Even high-intensity interval training—the kind of workout where people alternate periods of strenuous exercise with periods of rest—will only give you a couple of weeks of results before your body adapts. You'll get stronger, but you'll also get leaner and faster, and then…nothing.

Why? Because one way our bodies store energy is by enhancing its sensitivity to insulin, which helps it use fat as fuel. This adaptation is good for endurance activities like running or biking, since it helps your body get energy from stored fat. But it's not so good if you want to lose weight and burn body fat. The only way to overcome this adaptation is to keep increasing the intensity of your workouts—and that can spell trouble for your body.

The 15-minute workout works differently from traditional training because it takes advantage of what exercise scientists call the "pump effect" and "metabolic chaos": short bursts of intense activity followed by brief spurts of rest—all performed in 15 minutes or less. During and immediately after a workout, your body is flooded with stress hormones that boost your metabolism and increase fat burning. The 15-minute workout also keeps cortisol levels from spiking, which means you'll feel energized for hours after you exercise.

The 15-minute workout will give you a leaner, stronger body and a calmer mind—but it's important to realize that it won't give the same benefits as those long workouts you're used to. You won't see the same results in terms of strength and endurance because your body won't have enough time to adapt to the increased intensity. The good news is that most of this adaptation occurs in the first 15 minutes of your workout, and after that, you can just focus on having fun, getting healthier and feeling better.

The magic combination for the 15-minute workout is a mix of intense weight training and fast intervals of cardio. I have designed two different programs based on these principles—one for total-body leanness (which includes a full-body circuit) and one for building strength. Both use simple exercises you can do with a barbell for weight training, a pair of dumbbells at home or nothing more than your own body weight.

Chapter 1: The Science of 15-Minute Workouts

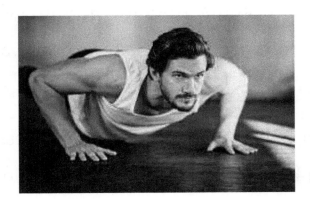

The best exercise, the most effective way to lose weight and get lean and healthy, takes place in the first 15 minutes of your workout. By "best" I mean that this type of workout is more effective than longer workouts because it boosts your body's metabolism and helps you burn fat. And by "least effective," I mean that workouts over an hour turn out to be counterproductive for most people, especially those who want to lose weight and build muscle. To be clear, this doesn't mean any exercise is better than no exercise. It just means that the kind of workout that offers the best results in the shortest period of time takes place in the first 15 minutes of your training sessions.

Advantages Over Traditional Workouts

1. It increases your metabolism and burns fat for hours after you exercise.

2. It keeps cortisol levels from spiking, which means you'll feel energized for hours after you exercise.

3. It's more effective in terms of building cardiovascular fitness than longer, less intense workouts (though if you get out of breath or lightheaded during your workouts, take a break and have a glass of water).

4. It leads to better weight loss than longer, less intense workouts because it helps you burn more fat in the hours following your workout (this point is debatable; see Chapter 7).

5. Your muscles respond positively to this type of workout with visible results; your body begins to shape up within two weeks.

6. It is more effective than longer, less intense workouts in terms of increasing muscle strength and endurance.

7. It keeps you focused on the workout itself, so you don't waste time worrying about what you're wearing or how much time the guy next to you lifts weights.

8. It's perfect for busy people who can't commit to longer exercise sessions (but even those who can devote an hour or more to their workout will benefit from including shorter sessions in their week).

9. It improves your mood and mental health because it boosts endorphins and helps reduce stress levels—even during a stressful day at the office.

Disadvantages Over Traditional Workouts

1. It is tough for beginners.

2. It takes up more time in your day than longer, less intense workouts do (though you can incorporate it into your busy life without much fuss).

3. It's not easy to stay motivated; you can feel like you're not doing enough in the beginning when your body is still adjusting to this type of training.

4. Some experts say shorter workouts aren't an effective way to build muscle, but the research I've cited tells a different story.

5. It can be very hard on your joints and spine.

6. It places a lot of stress on your body, which may lead to injury.

7. You're going to feel sore the next day (which is why this type of workout works best if you plan it for before work or on weekends).

8. You risk overtraining—doing too much too soon—which could leave you vulnerable to injury and burnout.

9. It might actually make weight loss harder because some studies show that working out intensely boosts your appetite.

10. Some people get bored doing shorter workouts, but you can switch up your routine to help stop this from happening.

11. You're more susceptible to skipping a workout or falling off the fitness wagon.

12. You may lack the energy to perform other activities in your day-to-day life, which is not what you want if you're trying to be healthy!

13. Some short workouts don't offer all of the health benefits that they claim (or any at all).

The most effective way to make sure you're benefiting from your workout regimen is to do workouts that are 30 minutes or longer. This is why an hour-long session at a gym, yoga studio, or fitness class works best - it takes about fifty minutes for your brain and body to be engaged enough to use the movements effectively while you're building endurance and strength. If you notice yourself struggling the first time you try something new, stick with it and don't give up until you can reap all of the benefits of the workout. And if you find yourself struggling with motivation, try pairing up with a friend! You can motivate each other; plus, research shows we work out more frequently when we have a buddy.

The length of your workout matters because it determines what is happening in your brain and body. Shorter workouts, even if they are intense, won't give you the same benefits as longer workouts. Even if you feel like you're getting leaner and stronger with your short workout, it could be that the change is not due to the workout improving your muscle tone or endurance - it might just be that your body is getting better at burning off fat and conserving energy.

You might think that some forms of exercise are more effective than others, but the duration of a workout is not what you should be focusing on. What really matters is that you participate in a workout that gets your heart rate up, improves your endurance and works your muscles. The type of training most people use to "get in shape" at gyms these days falls into two camps: interval training and resistance training. The problem with these two types of training is that they can be very hard on your body if performed too frequently over too long a duration. The interval training that fitness junkies are so fond of doesn't work for everyone—especially if you're new to the activity or have a bad hip. Resistance training is all about strength-building, which is why I designed the resistance program at FitnessBlueprint.com. It's one thing to get stronger, but why focus on it when endurance and fat-burning are your real goals? That's why I created a workout that focuses on fat burning and building muscular endurance without putting your body through hard intervals of cardio or stressful resistance training. To do it, you'll have to keep your heart rate up and your muscles working, but you don't have to put your body through tough intervals over and over again. The rest of this book will explain the science behind this exercise program—and how it can help you get leaner, stronger and fitter in just 15 minutes a day.

Chapter 2: Maximizing Your Weight-Training Workouts

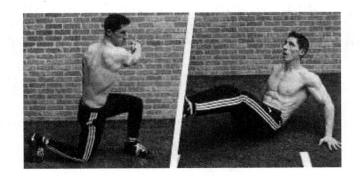

The best weight-training sessions last about 45 to 60 minutes, and they're designed to help you build lean muscle mass. Of course, that's not what we're going for. Our goal is to lose fat and improve our health, which is why I have designed a set of 15-minute workouts that will increase your metabolism and burn fat after each workout. These workouts are less intense than those traditional weight-training sessions that last an hour or more, and they don't require the same amount of time from you. You don't need to go to the gym and spend hours on exercise machines. You can lift weights using your own body weight, or you can use barbells and dumbbells you have at home. The workouts are simple, but that doesn't mean they're easy. To make them effective, you'll need to push yourself—and work through that discomfort you might feel if this is your first time doing a workout like this or if it has been a long time since you have done a good weight-training session. I designed this program to help build muscle mass using basic barbell exercises that work every muscle in your body - including your chest, back, shoulders, abs and legs. Your muscles will be responding to this type of training within two weeks, and you can expect that they will change in terms of appearance and performance. Not everyone wants to look like a bodybuilder, but most people want to look better. And this program—which takes place over just seven days—will help you do just that. You'll gain more muscle and lose more fat than you would with an hour-long, traditional workout. And even though this program is focused on building muscle, it will help you burn calories through the work your muscles do. It doesn't matter if you want to lose five pounds or 50—every workout you do shapes your body in some way. This program is for everyone because it uses compound exercises that work multiple muscles at once. If you are very out of shape, the 15-minute workouts will help you burn calories, improve your endurance and lift more than you ever have before. If you are already in good shape but want to get even stronger or more toned, this program will help. If your goal is to just build muscle and stay healthy, this is the program for you. Every workout will help you get stronger, which is what building muscle mass is all about. And you can expect to start noticing visible results within the first two weeks. Your muscles will be much firmer, your biceps will be more defined, your abs will be more pronounced and your legs will look leaner. If you already have some muscle mass or you spend the time to really work out those areas that need it, you can expect to see a difference in how your body looks in about six weeks. There is no such thing as spot reduction - where one area of your body (your butt, for example) gets smaller while another part (like your thighs) gets bigger - but this program does help promote lean muscle mass throughout the entire body. Every workout session burns calories and elevates the metabolism for hours after you've finished exercising. You'll also notice that your clothes fit better because you're leaner, and there will be fat burning 24/7.

This workout will help you create a calorie deficit - the difference between the calories you eat and the calories you burn off. The more time passes, the bigger that calorie deficit gets, which means you lose more weight faster. If your goal is to lose about 1 to 2 pounds per week, this workout will help you get there. Whether this is your first weight-training program or not, each session should feel just as intense as it does for someone who is just starting out at the gym. If you aren't feeling the burn or you are feeling fatigued, you are not pushing yourself hard enough. Push through your workouts. Every time you work out, you should be able to do more of the exercises than the last time.

Repeat each set of exercises twice. You can do each set back-to-back or rest 1 to 3 minutes in between before moving on to your next set. Rest 1 to 3 minutes between each round, and complete four rounds in total. Rest 1 day before moving on to the next workout session.

1. Chest Press

This exercise targets your pectoralis major, and it's a great way to build your chest if you are new to weight training or have been away from the gym for awhile. To do it, place a barbell on your upper back. You can use an Olympic bar or an EZ curl bar. Step underneath the bar and squat down low while holding onto its ends. Stand up straight while holding the bar with both hands at shoulder width.

2. Rear Deltoid Flyes

This is another great exercise for beginners because it doesn't require much knowledge about form or equipment. All you need is a bench and some dumbbells. Sit on the edge of the bench with your back facing the ceiling. Grab one dumbbell and rest it on your chest. Lower it out to the side while keeping your arms straight and elbows close to your body. Slowly bring it back up, squeeze your chest muscles and repeat for 10 reps on each side.

3. Triceps Dips

This exercise targets the triceps, which are some of the largest muscles in your upper arms. To do them, place a chair or bench so that it is standing behind you high enough that you can comfortably bend over and rest your weight on it without falling off. Place your hands on the edge of the bench with your fingers pointing towards you. Bend your legs under you and lower yourself until you feel a light stretch in your triceps. Press yourself back up, straighten your arms and repeat for 10 reps.

4. Dumbbell Curls

This exercise will help strengthen your biceps, which are the muscles in the front of your upper arms. Grab a set of light dumbbells - even a 2-pound set will work if that's all you have on hand at home - and stand with your feet shoulder-width apart. Keep your arms straight with a slight bend at the elbow, and lift them up towards your shoulders without moving them forward or back as you curl them up towards you chest. Squeeze your biceps at the top of the movement, and slowly bring them back to the starting position. Repeat for 8 to 10 reps.

5. Reverse Crunch

This exercise will help strengthen your core muscles, which are the ones in your abdomen and lower back. Lie on the floor with your knees bent up near your chest and feet flat on the ground. Place both hands behind your head or underneath your neck with elbows out (like you were going for an upside down push up). Lift yourself off of the ground by tightening in abs and pulling yourself up as if you were trying to touch your feet with your chest. Squeeze your abdominals as you exhale, and slowly lower yourself back down to the floor. Repeat for 10 reps.

6. One-Legged Dead Lift

This exercise will help strengthen your hamstrings and glutes, which are some of the largest muscles in the back of your legs. To do it, grab a barbell with a wide grip near the ends of its handle (but not so wide that it is hard to hold). Stand up straight with your feet shoulder-width apart and knees facing forward so that the barbell is hanging in front of you. Slowly bend at the waist while keeping your back straight and pulling down on the barbell with both hands until you feel a stretch in your hamstrings.

Chapter 3: Cardio and Mind-Body Training

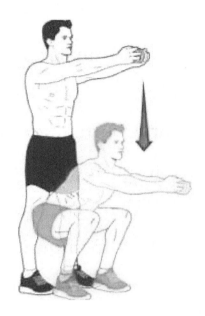

The best cardio workouts last about 45 to 60 minutes—and they can lead to a leaner body. That's how long it takes to get your heart rate up, burn calories and elevate the metabolism. That's also not what we're going for. Our goal here is to burn fat, which is why I have designed a set of 15-minute workouts that will help you access your fat stores and burn more fat after each workout. These workouts don't require the same amount of time from you because they aren't as intense as traditional cardio sessions that last an hour or more. But don't let that fool you—this isn't a light workout by any means. You will definitely feel them the next day because it takes a lot of work to burn calories and to build endurance. But the good thing is, you'll look forward to your workouts when they're over and you realize how much of a difference they are making in your life. This program will help you burn calories soon after each workout thanks to that calorie-burning effect called excess post-exercise oxygen consumption, or EPOC. You can think of EPOC as the afterburn effect, which makes it so that even after you are finished exercising, your body continues working for up to 24 hours after every workout session and burns more fat during that time. The only way to get this effect is to burn a lot of fat. The workouts in this program will help you do that. There are seven workout sessions in the program, and each one will last 15 minutes. I designed those short workouts to maximize your time and your results. They will help you burn calories and build endurance without being too intense or taking up too much time from your day. Each workout session uses a different cardio exercise so that you don't get bored from doing the same thing every day. Your muscles, joints and ligaments need rest in between exercises - especially if you are new to barbell training or resistance training in general. This program assumes that you are starting out with a basic understanding of how to lift weights, or that you have already gained enough control over your body and its movements to be able to complete the exercises safely. If you aren't sure if this program is right for you, talk with a certified trainer or fitness professional who can help you decide whether or not it is a good fit for your current fitness level.

To get the most out of this workout plan, do each session 2 or 3 times per week. You can do it every other day, but I would recommend spacing them out by at least two days so that your muscles have some time to repair themselves between training sessions. If you are just starting out, you might want to choose a lighter exercise session for days when you are doing your upper body workout. If you aren't sure which workout session is right for your fitness level, talk with a certified trainer or fitness professional who can help you decide.

1. Bodyweight Squats

This is a great way to warm up before your workout. It's not only good for building strength and increasing flexibility, it also burns calories. Stand with your feet shoulder-width apart and hold your arms out in front of you at shoulder height with palms facing down. Lean your weight back into your heels, and lower yourself towards the ground while flexing your knees to 90 degrees. Keep going until you feel a light stretch in your calves or thighs, then press back up and repeat for 50 reps.

2. Pushups

This is another great workout to do as a warm-up. Pushups are a compound exercise that work out your chest, abs and shoulders, and they also help strengthen your triceps and biceps. To do them, lie facedown with your hands spread out about shoulder-width apart underneath you. Lower yourself towards the ground until your chest nearly touches it while keeping your elbows at 90 degrees. Press yourself back up to the starting position by pushing with your arms, shoulders and chest. Repeat for 50 reps.

3. Lunge Jumps With Pushup

This is a bodyweight exercise that will definitely get you sweating! To do it, start in a standing position with feet shoulder-width apart and hands on hips. Step forward with one foot about two and a half feet out from your body, and bend both knees until you feel a light stretch in your thigh. Your back knee should be nearly touching the ground, but keep it just an inch off the ground without letting it touch. Press yourself back up to the starting position by pushing with your front leg muscles, then jump up as high as you can and land softly on the ground in the same position you were in when you started. Repeat for 15 reps on each leg.

4. Skaters

This is another compound exercise that will get your heart pumping! To do this exercise, stand with feet shoulder-width apart and arms out at your sides with palms facing forward. Jump up and down on your toes, and move your arms back and forth in a running motion while you jump. The faster you are moving your arms, the easier it will be to get your heart rate up. Repeat for 25 jumps.

5. Leg Lifts

This exercise is great for toning and strengthening your lower abdominal area! Start lying on the floor with legs together and arms at your sides with palms facing down. Raise both legs off the ground as high as you can by bringing in both the front and back sides of both legs. Squeeze those same muscles on the way back down to the starting position, then repeat for 15 reps.

6. Walking Lunges

This bodyweight exercise is one of my favourites - it exercises so many different muscles at once! Stand with your feet shoulder-width apart and arms out in front of you at shoulder height with palms facing down. Step forward with one foot about two and a half feet out from your body, and bend both knees until you feel a light stretch in your thigh. Your back knee should be nearly touching the ground, but keep it just an inch off the ground without letting it touch. Press yourself back up to the starting position by pushing with your front leg muscles, then jump up as high as you can and land softly on the ground in the same position you were in when you started. Step forward with your other leg, then repeat for 15 reps on each leg.

7. Burpees

This is another compound exercise that will get your heart pumping! Burpees are a full body exercise that burn a lot of calories and strengthen all of the major muscles in your body, including your arms, shoulders, back and chest. To do them, start standing up straight with feet shoulder-width apart and hands on hips or at shoulder height with palms facing down. Jump up as high as you can towards the ceiling by pushing from both legs and throwing both arms straight out in front of you. Press yourself back up to the starting position by bending at the knees and hips, then immediately jump into the air again and repeat for 15 reps.

8. Side Knee Lifts

This is another exercise that is great for toning your lower abdominal area! Start lying on a side with one leg straight out in front of you and the other bent at a 90 degree angle with foot flat on the ground. The bottom foot can be flat or you can lift it off of the ground slightly. Lift you top knee as high as you can towards your chest while keeping your hips up, then lower it back down to the starting position. Repeat for 50 reps, then switch sides and repeat with your other leg.

9. Mountain Climbers

This is another full body exercise that will get your heart pumping! Start out in a push-up position with back straight and feet together. With one leg, step forward so that your knee comes up to your chest while you are still in the push-up position. When you bring your knee back down to the floor, switch legs and repeat on that side. Repeat for 15 reps, then switch sides and repeat with your other leg.

10. Plank Jumps

This bodyweight exercise is an excellent workout for strengthening both of your arms since the resistance comes from holding yourself up! To do it, lie face down with upper torso off of the floor so that you are resting on forearms and toes. Hold yourself up as long as you can, then jump up and land softly on the floor. Repeat for 15 jumps.

11. Plank Holds

This exercise will help strengthen your core muscles and keep your body toned! To do it, lie face down on the floor with legs together and arms at your sides with palms facing down. Raise both legs off the ground as high as you can by bringing in both the front and back sides of both legs without dropping either of your shoulders or hips to the floor while holding yourself up with forearms and toes. Hold that position as long as you can, then lower yourself back to the starting position by slowly lowering both arms, feet and hips to the ground before repeating for 3 minutes.

Cardio Workouts are great because they get your heart rate up and help you stay focused during each exercise session. The key to success is to make sure you find a plan that will work for your body and your current fitness level. You should be able to push yourself each time you exercise, but you should also make sure that the exercises are challenging enough to allow room for progress when you return to that routine again. Only by pushing yourself will you see results, so find a workout plan that is right for you and start seeing changes today!

Cardio Workouts are great because they get your heart rate up and help you stay focused during each exercise session. The key to success is to make sure you find a plan that will work for your body and your current fitness level. You should be able to push yourself each time you exercise, but you should also make sure that the exercises are challenging enough to allow room for progress when you return to that routine again. Only by pushing yourself will you see results, so find a workout plan that is right for you and start seeing changes today!

This program is a perfect example of how getting in shape doesn't have to be hard or boring! If you currently don't have any workout routines, this plan has all of the tools and suggestions you need to get started on your path towards a healthier life.

Chapter 4: 15-Minute Training Plans

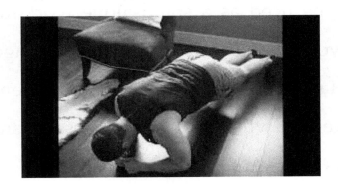

Cardio Workouts are great because they get your heart rate up and help you stay focused during each exercise session. The key to success is to make sure you find a plan that will work for your body and your current fitness level. You should be able to push yourself each time you exercise, but you should also make sure that the exercises are challenging enough to allow room for progress when you return to that routine again. Only by pushing yourself will you see results, so find a workout plan that is right for you and start seeing changes today! These 15-minute training plans can be used for aerobic workouts or resistance training. They are all great if you have little time in your day but want a quick, effective workout.

1. The 5-Minute Workout If you are really short on time and want to get an intense workout in, then this program is perfect for you. It's a great way to get your muscles pumping and to start sweating with just a few minutes of exercising!

2. The 10-Minute Workout This workout plan is easy and quick, yet still gets results! It can be used as a stand-alone workout plan or as extra cardio work after you have already performed a longer training session on another day. Many people find that it helps them lose weight and stay focused on exercise when they do this less intensive training after their long workouts are over for the week.

3. The 15-Minute Workout This full-body training program will get your heart pumping in just fifteen short minutes! It's a great way to get your body warmed up and ready for more intense workouts later in the week.

4. The 30-Minute Workout Many people find that they have time to exercise in the mornings before work, but if you have trouble keeping yourself motivated in the mornings, then this program is for you! This routine is designed to be done right after waking up so that it doesn't interfere with your breakfast or morning routine.

5. 30-Minute Upper Body Workout Whether you are trying to impress the ladies or just want to look good shirtless, this workout plan will give you the muscles you're looking for in just thirty minutes! This program is perfect for everyone - men, women and even children.

6. The 30-Minute Full Body Workout This full body training program is great for building muscle and increasing endurance. It's a perfect

training plan to help you get into shape after a long break from working out or if you want to train more intensely than usual.

7. The 30-Minute Lower Body Workout If you want to really build muscle in your biceps, quads and calves, then this is the training plan for you. It's a great way to train all of the muscles in your lower body if you are trying to improve your overall strength or if you want to increase the muscle on a specific part of your body.

8. The 30-Minute Upper & Lower Body Workout This workout program is designed specifically for people who want to work on both their upper and lower body with equal intensity at the same time! It's a great training plan that will tone and strengthen your muscles while also working on mobility and endurance.

Full body program that uses both free weights and exercise machines to tone and strengthen your entire body. This workout plan is great for people who want to focus on building muscle or toning their entire body with just fifteen minutes of exercising each day. This training plan will get your heart pumping and help you burn fat all over your body! It's also great as a supplement to other training programs, so use it as an extra workout after you have already put in a longer training session. It's never too late to start becoming the best version of yourself!

This stand-alone workout plan is designed specifically for people who want to work on their upper body and nothing else. If you currently lift weights or do other exercises to build your muscles, then this workout plan can be added on after you have finished a longer training session that works on areas other than your arms, shoulders, chest and back. It's a great way to increase the intensity of your training sessions if you find yourself too tired or short on time for a longer workout later in the week. Use it alone or as an extra workout after you have completed a longer training routine on another day.

This bodyweight training program uses various muscles in your body to tone and strengthen your muscles. It's great for quick workouts that don't take too long but will still give you the results you are looking for! This program is also great for kids who want to keep their bodies healthy while they are growing up. This bodyweight training program is great for getting in shape without taking up your precious time! It's a great way to stay fit when you are travelling, working late or if you just have very little time for exercising. It will help keep your muscles strong and improve your endurance while helping you burn fat all over your body.

Endurance is essential for staying healthy and strong throughout the years. If you want to train your body to be able to run fast and far, then this program is perfect for you! It's designed to be a long distance training plan that will help you run faster and farther than ever before by increasing your endurance. It's perfect for people who already have experience running or prefer not to use weight training programs. This program will help you tone and strengthen your muscles while also building up the muscles in your legs. The best way to improve the strength of your legs is by increasing the amount of weight that they are lifting, so this program does just that!

This high intensity interval training (HIIT) workout plan is great for people who want a quick workout with high intensity. Your heart rate will be elevated for the entire workout plan, so this is a great way to burn fat and keep yourself in shape! It's also perfect for people who want to increase the intensity of their workouts but don't have much time to work out. Remember that you should only do this workout 2-3 times a week, as it is intense and will take its toll on your body if you do it more often.

Chapter 5: The Top 10 Motivators to Work Out for 15 Minutes or Less

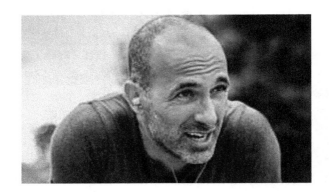

Are you looking for some motivation to get your workout on? If you need a little extra push to get up and start exercising, then look no further. This chapter will provide you with the motivation and tools you need to get moving today! Motivation plays an important part in your ability to stay fit and healthy, so make sure that you have the proper motivation before heading out into the world for a run or a workout at the gym. This chapter will also give you some great tips on how to stay motivated when working out can be hard. These are all great ways that top athletes use to keep themselves motivated on days when they think they can't go on. When you're looking for a little motivation, remember that these athletes are regular people who use these techniques to push themselves harder. It may not work for everyone, but it's worth a shot! Here are the top ten motivators to get you started:

1. Exercise with Someone Who Keeps You Motivated Whether you are going to a class or working out alone at the gym, make sure you find someone who will keep you motivated throughout your workout. Working out with a friend can make workouts more enjoyable and will keep you pushing yourself until the very end.

2. Do Something You Love Sometimes exercising can be hard if it feels like a chore that doesn't make any sense to do in the first place. If you are looking for a way to make working out more fun, then try finding something you love to do that gets your heart racing. Maybe you like a certain sport, or maybe just jogging outside is what makes you happy. If there's something that makes your heart pump and your body move, then use it as a motivator to push yourself harder!

3. Set a Goal to Meet Sometimes it's easy to lose sight of why we're doing this in the first place. If you are looking for some motivation, then create a specific goal for yourself that will keep you on the right track towards success. If you want to lose weight, then keep that goal in mind every time you exercise and it will keep you focused on your success.

4. Plan a Specific Time for Working Out If you are looking for motivation, then the best way to stay motivated is to plan a specific time that you can work out. This is especially helpful if you have trouble staying motivated or getting up early in the morning. Even if it's just 5

minutes a day, planning specific times can help get your body moving even when you don't think you can.

5. Think About What You Could Do Without It Sometimes it's hard to understand what we have until we lose it altogether. If you are having trouble getting motivated, then think about what you would be missing if you weren't able to work out. What would your life be like if you hated going to the gym? Would your clothes fit right? Would your health be in danger? Would you look physically different with all of that extra weight on your body?

6. See Yourself at a Specific Weight When working out, sometimes it's easy to forget how far you have come and what your goal is in the first place. If you see a great picture of yourself looking fit and healthy, then use it as motivation to keep going when things start getting tough. It will remind you of your original goal and keep you on the right track to success.

7. Listen to Motivating Music There are lots of ways to get motivated in the world today, and one of them is listening to music that makes you want to move! Music with a strong beat and energizing lyrics can really push you harder during your workout. Some people find it hard to get into a rhythm when exercising without music while others think it takes away from their workout, but no matter what, listening to specific songs can be great motivation when working out.

8. Focus on What You Have Already Achieved Working out is all about achieving as much as we possibly can. Sometimes it's easy to forget how far we have come with our workouts, but if you are having trouble getting motivated, then think about what you have already accomplished. Maybe you ran a mile this week or maybe your muscles look a little more toned. Think about everything that you have already done and use that as motivation to continue on the right track towards success.

9. Focus on What You Are Doing While Working Out Sometimes it can be hard to motivate yourself when working out because you don't feel like working out in the first place! If you are finding yourself lacking motivation, then try focusing on what your body is doing while exercising rather than focusing on actually doing the workout itself. This will help you stay focused and keep your motivation on the right track.

10. Use a Workout Buddy Having a workout buddy can be extremely helpful if you are looking for some extra motivation to get you through your workout plan. If you have someone to exercise with, then make sure that they are serious about their workouts so that they can push you harder! It may also help if they are trying to do the same thing as you – whether that is losing weight or getting stronger – than working

out with them will be a great way to reach your goal faster than ever before.

Chapter 6: The 15-Minute Workout Log

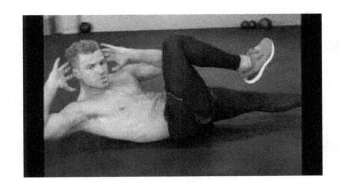

Keep track of your workouts with the workout log! This chapter will show you how to log your workouts for fifteen minutes or less. You will be able to keep track of your daily progress and create a custom workout plan that will keep you at a specific heart rate. This chapter will also give you some tips on how to make sure that your heart rate is right throughout each exercise. Depending on the workout program that you are using, it can be difficult to know exactly when to stop exercising during your training session. There are various ways to monitor this, but one of the best ways is using a heart rate monitor. It is most accurate if you have a heart rate monitor that works with your Smartphone, but it can also be used with free apps on your phone. This way, you can make sure that your heart stays in the right range and doesn't get too high or too low while working out. This is also great because it allows you to monitor your heart rate while running or exercising outside. If you plan on running, then make sure that your heart rate is monitored and stay in the correct heart rate zone. If you are looking for a quick way to monitor your heart rate, then you can always use a free app on your phone or hear rate monitor that is designed for high intensity workouts.

These are some of the best ways to keep track of your fitness:

1: The Basic Log This is probably one of the most common ways to track your workout. If you want something simple and easy to use, then this might be the best way for you. It's great because it's simple and it works! All you have to do is record basic information, such as the date and time, what you did during your workout, how long it took and maybe some additional notes about how it went. Record this in a notebook, on your computer or if you are using an app, then use that to log the information.

2: The Calorie Log If you are looking to lose weight, then this might be the log for you. This will help you keep track of your calories burned throughout the day and it will also tell you exactly how many calories you've burned during each workout session. This helps because it will keep track of everything for you and make sure that your fitness routine is working. It will also help to encourage you if things start getting tough because it will show how much progress you have made so far.

3: The Custom Log Depending on which fitness routine you are using, you might want to create a custom log. This way, you can keep track of everything that you should be doing and make sure that your body is getting what it needs. If there are certain exercises that you know your body needs, then make sure that those exercises are getting done! Use a spreadsheet or contact paper as a way to track your progress.

4: The Simple Log If you are looking for something simple and easy to use, then this might be the best choice for you. This will help keep track of some basic information and provide a little structure so that you know exactly how to keep track of your workouts. However, if you are using this log and you want more of a challenge, then try adding some extra exercises that you can do during your workout.

5: The Specific Log If you are looking for something simple and easy to use, but also want to keep track of your heart rate throughout the entire workout, then this might be the log for you. It has been designed specifically for workouts that last around fifteen minutes or less. All you have to do is follow the recommended heart rate zone that works best for your body and then record it throughout the workout. This way, you will know exactly what your heart rate should be at any given moment during the workout session.

6: The Workout Log Keeping track of your workouts is important whether you're training for a competition or just looking to get healthier and more fit. However, it can be a challenge to figure out what information you should be keeping track of and which information isn't necessary. This type of log will allow you to keep track of exactly how you are doing and how many calories you've burned during each workout session. It also keeps an accurate record of your heart rate zones so that you can make sure that your heart stays in the right range for the entire duration of the workout.

Chapter 7: The Equipment You Need

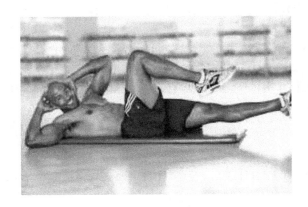

If you are going to be working out at home, then you will need a few pieces of equipment to really get the most out of your fitness routine. You don't have to have a lot of equipment in order to workout and be successful, but it would be ideal if you could find some good quality equipment that is easy for you to use. This chapter will show you the best types of equipment for using at home and how much each item costs.

The Best Equipment for Home Use

1: Two 5-pound dumbbells If you are just starting out and looking for something simple that won't cost much, then 5-pound dumbbells might be the right choice for you. These are usually the least expensive and can help you get in shape by using them for basic exercises. If you are looking for something to work your arms and shoulders, then these will be a great choice.

2: Two or Three 10-pound dumbbells If you are looking for something stronger than 5-pound weights, then 10-pound weights might be a better option for you. These will help build your strength and endurance much faster and are also good for working out your arms and shoulders.

3: One 25-pound dumbbell If you are looking to start lifting heavier weights, then this might be the best choice for you. This is also a good weight for working out your shoulders and arms.

4: A 10-pound medicine ball If you are looking to add some variety to your weight lifting routine, then a medicine ball will be a great choice for you. These are great for working out your upper body and building strength in your core. They can also help you improve balance and stability if you throw them around while working out.

5: A foam roller Foam rollers are a relatively new piece of equipment that have come about over the last few years of fitness training. If you have never tried one, then they can help relieve pain in your muscles after exercising or running long distances.

6: A weighted jump rope If you want to get a good jump rope, then this might be the best choice for you. These ropes come in various weights, but they are great for increasing your cardio and building up endurance. They are also really fun to use!

7: A jump mat This is another great choice and will help you stay safe while doing basic exercises like sit-ups or push-ups. These mats can also help decrease the risk of injury while doing cardio workouts.

8: Resistance bands If you need something to work your legs out without stepping on a treadmill or run outside, then resistance bands might be the right choice for you. These come in various sizes and are great for targeting specific muscles.

Finding the Best Equipment for Home Use If you are looking to purchase any of these items, then look online at stores like Target or Amazon, or try a local sports equipment store. Make sure that the equipment is high quality and will last you a long time. They should also be easy to use and should be able to help you reach your workout goals in no time!

Chapter 8: The Healthiest Foods on Earth: Super foods to Fuel Your 15-Minute Workouts and Other Health Longer.

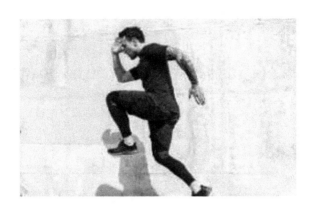

This is a list of some of the healthiest foods on earth, as well as what they can do for you. These are great to have in your fridge, so make sure that you grab something healthy to eat after a hard workout session.

7 Food Superstars for Healthy Hearts Heart disease is one of the most common causes of death in America, but there are ways to keep your heart healthy. One of the best ways to do this is by eating healthy foods. These are the healthiest foods that you can eat for your heart and some of them may surprise you.

1: Grapefruit This crispy fruit is full of nutrients and vitamins that are good for your heart and blood vessels. They also have a lot of potassium in them, which helps lower blood pressure and reduce risk of stroke. If you're feeling like your heart isn't getting enough attention, then grapefruit might be a great way to help!

2: Avocados Remember these from your favourite guacamole? They actually have a ton of health benefits because they are filled with omega-3 fatty acids, vitamin E, vitamin C and potassium. They are also good for preventing coronary heart disease and cardiac arrest.

3: Oatmeal It might be common knowledge that oatmeal is good for your diet, but did you know that it is also great for your heart? It is full of soluble fibber which can help lower cholesterol and blood sugar levels.

4: Herring If you were looking to eat something savoury, then this might be what you're looking for! Herring has omega-3 fatty acids which help to reduce cholesterol and triglyceride levels in the blood. These are also great if you have a hard time eating leafy greens or other vegetables because they can be added to almost any dish.

5: Salmon Salmon is another fish that is great for your heart. It is full of omega-3 fatty acids and vitamin D, which are both important for reducing the risk of heart disease. This fish also has enough Omega-6 Omega-3 fatty acids to help your body absorb more fat and prevent heart disease and high blood pressure.

6: Tomatoes Remember to eat the skin because it may not be as healthy as you think! These bad boys are low in calories, but high in lycopene and antioxidants. They also have lots of fibre to help keep you full longer and improve digestion.

7: Beans These are one of those healthy foods that you probably remember from your childhood. They are great for heart health because they have lots of fibre, protein and potassium in them. If you don't like black beans, then you can try out some pinto beans or kidney beans as a way to help your heart stay healthy.

The Best Foods for Your Heart If you want to be sure that your heart is staying strong and healthy, then consider adding some of these foods to your diet. Eating healthy gives your body what it needs to stay healthy and also avoids some of the diseases that plague people every day.

The Best Foods for Your Brain

3 Super Foods for Focused Thinking and Improved Memory

If you want to keep your mind sharp and your memory intact, then you need to make sure that you are eating healthy foods. This focuses on three foods that are great for maintaining focus while exercising or just trying to get through work. These super foods also improve memory and can help keep your mind sharp while giving you a fun boost of energy when you need it most.

1: Walnuts This is a great source of omega-3 fatty acids and antioxidants that help to protect your brain from age-related memory loss. These nuts also contain lots of vitamin E, which is great for learning and memory.

2: Avocado Peppers This might be one of the most delicious super foods out there, but did you know that it is also full of good fats that can improve memory? It has vitamin B6 in it as well, which helps regulate blood sugar levels.

3: Wild Blueberries Blueberries are one of the healthiest fruits on earth and they come packed with nutrients that are good for your brain. These berries are also full of vitamin C, which helps to reduce stress and improve focus. If you eat a handful of these berries before a workout or before work, then you will be giving your body and mind the boost that it needs.

The Best Foods for Your Brain If you want to exercise your mind as well as your body, then consider eating any of these super foods on a regular basis. Those who eat healthy live longer and tend to have fewer health issues than those who don't!

The Best Foods for Your Colon

3 Super Foods for Happy Digestion

Your digestive system is responsible for absorbing nutrients from all the food in your diet. It needs to be healthy to get all the nutrients that you need, but it can also be affected by stress and illness. This will teach you about three foods that are great for improving digestion and keeping your colon in good shape!

1: Broccoli This might be a familiar vegetable, but did you know that it is great for your colon? It has lots of fibre, potassium and vitamin C in it, which are all essential in keeping your digestive system moving the right way.

2: Parsley Did you know that parsley is actually healthy? It is full of antioxidants and fibre that can help prevent bad stomach problems like constipation or diarrhoea. These are great for people who experience bloating or indigestion regularly.

3: Beans Beans are one of the healthiest foods on earth and they are full of fibre that will help clean out your colon. They also have lots of protein in them, which helps to regulate your stomach and improve digestion.

The Best Foods for Your Colon If you want to stay regular and happy, then consider eating any of these super foods on a regular basis. If you regularly have problems with bloating or indigestion, then this can help you regulate your stomach and get rid of the bloated feeling.

Chapter 9: The 15-Minute Mind-Body Workout Plan for a Better Brain and a Calmer You

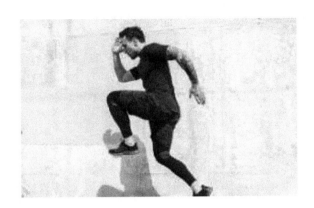

This is a sample workout plan that can be used for working on your brain or body. You should be able to do this at home with very little equipment and it only takes 15 minutes! Just get yourself ready and go over the plan to see how you can work out your body in just 15 minutes. This is easier than you think!

1. 2-3 Warm Up Exercises This will help loosen up your muscles before you do the rest of the workout. Try walking for 3 minutes and then stretch your arms, legs, back and shoulders before you attack the rest of your workout.

2. 3-4 Strength Exercises These exercises will help build up your muscles and start to burn calories. Do each exercise for around 30 seconds and then take a short break before you move on to the next one.

3. 2-3 Cool Down Exercises If you are looking for something to cool down your body, then use the next few exercises to stretch out your muscles and get loose again. Try sitting down in a chair with your legs stretched out in front of you and lean back with one hand behind your head. This will help improve flexibility in your shoulders and hips.

4. 2-3 Stretching Exercises If you want to get even more flexible, then try three more stretches for your hips, legs and arms. Hold each stretch for around 30 seconds and then roll your shoulders and neck to loosen them.

5. 3-4 Breathing Exercises These breathing exercises are great for calming your mind and preparing you to finish the workout. They will also help regulate your heartbeat as well as boost energy levels. To do these exercises, breathing in through your nose for 3 counts and hold it in for 3 counts. Slowly exhale for 6 counts before taking a deep breath again.

6. 2-3 Deep Breathing Exercises You should also try out some deep breathing exercises at the end of the workout to help you relax. Breathing in through your nose for 5 counts and slowly exhale for 10 counts. Repeat this 6 times to get rid of stress and relax.

7. 2-3 Meditation Exercises If you want something a little more challenging, then meditation exercises are a great way to finish the workout. Sit down with your back straight, close your eyes and focus on your breathing for two minutes. This will help keep you relaxed and focused before continuing on with the rest of your day.

8. 2-3 Cool Down Exercises If you want to stretch out your muscles after the workout, then be sure to do it using the next few exercises. Try sitting in a chair with your legs outstretched in front of you and lean back with one hand behind your head. This will help improve flexibility in your hips and shoulders.

9. 3-4 Breathing Exercises You can also try out these breathing exercises at the end of the workout to help you relax further. Breathing in through your nose for 3 counts and hold it in for 3 counts. Slowly exhale through your mouth for 6 counts before taking a deep breath again.

Chapter 10: The 15-Minute Exercises You Can Do Anywhere

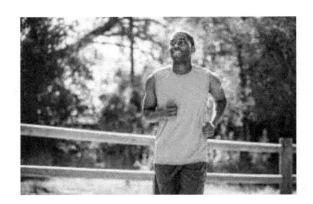

Did you know that you can do a workout without a gym? It's true! You can do it almost anywhere and with the right exercises, you can get in shape in less than 15 minutes. This is the best part of all because it doesn't matter where you are when your body needs to be exercised. Here are some of the best exercises that you can try out.

1. 2-3 Warm Up Exercises Warming up before your workout is one of the most important things that you need to do and it only takes about 5 minutes for this. You should start off by walking for 2 minutes and then stretch your arms, shoulders, legs and back for another minute. When you feel ready to move on, then you can jump right into the workout.

2. 3-4 Strength Exercises Pick 3 different exercises for your body and do each one for 1 minute before taking a break. You should try squats,

lunges and pushups at first to work out your core as well as your legs. You can also try arm raises to work out your arms.

3. 3-4 Cool Down Exercises After you are done with the strength exercises, then use the next few minutes to cool down with some more stretching and breathing exercises. Try sitting in a chair with your legs extended in front of you and lean back while resting one hand behind your head.

4. 2-3 Stretching Exercises After you have cooled down, then be sure to do some more stretching for your arms, legs and shoulders. You should also roll your neck and shoulders to loosen them up. If you want to take the best care of your body, then you should try out these exercises so that you can get back in shape in a safe and effective way!

5. 2-3 Breathing Exercises These exercises are great for relaxing your body and helping it to stay calm throughout the day. To do them, breathe in through your nose for 5 counts before holding it in for 10 counts. Slowly exhale through your mouth for 8 counts before taking another deep breath. This helps to reduce stress and calm your body down.

6. 2-3 Deep Breathing Exercises This is one of the hardest parts of any workout, but it's important that you try them out! To do these

exercises, breath in through your nose for 5 counts and slowly exhale through your mouth for 10 counts. Repeat this 6 times to help relax your body and mind.

7. 2-3 Meditation Exercises These are the most difficult exercises of all because they take a lot of focus to do correctly. If you want something more challenging, then sit in a chair with your back straight, close your eyes and focus on breathing for 2 minutes. This will help keep you relaxed and focused whenever you need to be.

8. 3-4 Breathing Exercises You can also try out these breathing exercises at the end of your workout to help you relax. Breath in through your nose for 4 counts and hold it in for 5 counts. Slowly exhale through your mouth for 8 counts before taking a deep breath again.

9. 2-3 Cool Down Exercises If you want to stretch out your muscles, then use the next few minutes to try some basic stretching exercises for your shoulders, arms and legs. This will help stretch out any tight muscles from the workout as well as loosen up tight joints that make it hard to move around easily.

10. 2-3 Stretching Exercises If you want to do a little more, then try some more stretching exercises for your arms, legs and shoulders. You should also roll your neck and shoulders to loosen them up and improve flexibility.

Chapter 11: A New You in Just 15 Minutes.

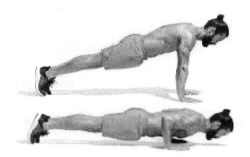

If you follow the workout plan in this book and eat healthy, then you will start to see a difference in your body and health. Your body will be happier, stronger and more flexible than ever before. This is how:

Eating Healthy You might have heard that eating healthy is the best way to improve your health, but do you know how it works? The food that we put into our bodies has to be able to digest easily so that we can absorb all of the nutrients that we need. If the food does not digest well, then it will go through your colon and get trapped there for a long time. This will cause your colon to become sluggish and fat deposits will build up behind the stool. Over time, your colon will get bigger and bigger because your body is not getting the nutrients that it needs. Your digestive system will eventually get blocked because it can no longer push the stool through your colon and out of your body. If you constantly eat foods that are hard to digest, then you will have to deal with serious lifestyle issues in the future. This is why you need to change your diet and start eating more vegetables and fruits instead of processed foods. You will also want to stop drinking soda or alcohol if you currently do. These drinks are full of sugar, which is hard for your body to absorb if you don't have enough fibre in your diet. Your digestive system needs fibres so that it can get rid of the unabsorbed food. If you are trying to lose weight, then focus on eating more vegetables and fruits. This will help you to get rid of excess water and boost your metabolism at the same time. You should also avoid fried foods because they are high in fat as well as saturated fats that will stick to the walls of your colon. You need to avoid this because it will make your body start to swell up and cause digestive problems like constipation, bloating or diarrhoea. Fiber is also very important for keeping a healthy digestive system and you can get it by eating lots of green leafy vegetables, oatmeal, oat bran, wheat bran and whole grains. Over time, you will see a huge difference in your digestive health and you should start to have much less constipation and bloating. Your body will no longer hold onto excess water or get impacted by extra pounds. You can also add some probiotic yogurt into your diet because it contains good bacteria that helps break down food so that it can be digested. This is very helpful for those that have digestive issues like diarrhoea because the good bacteria restores balance to their intestines after being sick or drinking certain beverages.

3-4 Minutes of Exercise Doing a few minutes of exercise every day will improve the way that your body moves. You will start to feel stronger, more flexible and much more relaxed. In fact, it only takes around 3 minutes of exercise to realize some of the health benefits which is why you should add 15 minutes into your busy schedule every day. Since you can do this in your own home or office, there are no excuses not to do it! When it comes to moving your body around, then try out some squats with weights and lunges. You should also try going for a walk around the block or even running up and down flights of stairs if you have the time. If you want to get even more movement in your body, then you should try out some yoga poses every day. You can do the sun salutation stretch or do some of the simpler moves like downward facing dog or child's pose.

3-4 Minutes of Breathing Exercises It is also important that you take the time to focus on breathing exercises that will help you to calm down and relax. You should try three different breathing exercises every day for at least 3 minutes each. Try out the diaphragmatic breath, corpse pose and box breathing exercise so that you can clear your mind and relax your body.

3-4 Minutes of Deep Breathing Exercises The most important thing that you can do is to practice deep breathing every day for a few minutes. This will help you to relax and calm down when you are feeling stressed or anxious. You should practice breathing exercises by sitting in a chair with your back straight and then breathe in through your nose for 5 counts before slowly exhaling through your mouth for 10 counts. Repeat this 6 times so that you can start to clear your mind and relax.

2-3 Minutes of Meditation Exercises If you want something that is a little more challenging, then focus on practicing meditation exercises every day for 2 to 3 minutes. This will help you to feel happy and relaxed for the rest of your day. You should sit somewhere comfortable with your back straight before closing your eyes and focusing on breathing for 2 minutes. This is a great way to get in a relaxed state and focus on the good things in your life as well as forget about everything else!

The Benefits Of Working Out In A Group

If you are trying to lose weight or get into shape, then you might be wondering whether it's better to do these things alone or with a group of friends. In fact, you can do both because each method has its own advantages and disadvantages. Here are some reasons as to why you might want to join a group in the future.

3-4 Reasons To Work Out In A Group

1. Accountability When you work out in a group, then it is easy to get distracted or start talking about other things that are going on in your

life. This is why it's important for everyone to hold each other accountable so that they can be sure that the workout will happen as planned and nothing else will come up. When everyone is working out together, then no one wants to let the other people down by not being there or doing exercises incorrectly.

2. Motivation If you are suffering from motivation issues, then you should join a group so that you can enjoy the fun of working out with your friends.

3. Healthy Competition Working out in a group will also help you to have healthy competition to keep your body motivated and moving in the right way. You should always expect to get the best results if you are working out with other people because this will encourage everyone to stay on track. It's important for everyone to keep each other accountable so that everyone succeeds together and it's not just one person that gets healthier while others go back to eating unhealthy foods or giving up on their goals.

4 Things To Do When Joining A Group

a. Try Out Different Workout Classes There are so many workout classes available for you to choose from, so it can be hard to know where to start. Luckily, you can try out different classes until you find one that matches your fitness level and goals. You should try out a class that is something new to you every few weeks so that you get the most benefits possible.

b. Check Your Level Of Skill If the rules of the class are too hard for you, then talk to your instructor about working at a different skill level or coming back again when your skills have improved. It's a terrible feeling to attend a high-level class when you are not ready to do the exercises yet, so talk to the instructor if you have any skill or ability issues.

c. Get To Know The Skill Of Other People One of the most important things that you can do is work out with other people that are at your skill level so that you can encourage each other to stay motivated and get better results over time. You should also talk to the others about what they like most about working out in a group and how they enjoy motivating each other on social media.

d. Workout With Other People For Accountability Having someone to work out with for accountability is very important and you should definitely invite your friends to join you as well. If they already work out, then it will be easy to go at the same time and do the same exercises. You can even take turns encouraging each other as you workout so that no one gets distracted by their surroundings or weakens when they are having a bad time.

3-4 Things To Avoid When Working Out in a Group

1. Obsessing Over Weight If you are truly working out with other people for motivation, then you should know that they are focused on their own results more than yours. If they want to lose weight, then they will follow their own program and it might be different from your workout plan so don't let this bother you. You can check out the same workout plan that your friend is following so that you push each other to stay accountable.

2. Spreading Bad Energy If you can't help but be negative about your workout or results, then don't bother joining a group. You will only end up spreading bad energy to others and they will lose faith in their fitness program.

3. Not Staying Safe If you are trying to work out in a group, then it's important to make sure that everyone is staying safe at all times throughout the exercises so that no one gets injured. If you see that someone is doing something wrong, then point it out and see if they can correct their form so that they don't get hurt.

4. Not Getting Results You should also be aware that it might be a little harder to get results when you are working out in a group because you aren't sure what might affect your results. It's important for everyone to follow the same workout schedule so that everyone gets the results that they want over time.

The Benefits Of Yoga In a Mat

Yoga in a mat is a great exercise to try out because it will help you to have more flexibility, a stronger core and better balance. You should add this exercise to your workout schedule if you are looking for something new and low impact so that you can get the best results possible. To do this, follow these instructions.

1. Sitting Position The first step is to sit down on a soft mat with your legs crossed and your hands in your lap. You want to either have the palms facing up or the fingers pointing toward the top of your head before you begin breathing exercises.

2. Breathing Exercises Next, you need to focus on your breathing by doing a breathing exercise for 3-4 minutes. You should breathe in for 5 counts before exhaling for 10 counts. You can practice this note breathing exercise for about 6 times to start feeling more relaxed and calm.

3. Lying Position Next, you need to lie down on your back before taking the time to focus on your breathing for 2 minutes. You should close your eyes and focus on breathing in for 5 counts before breathing out for 10 counts. This is a great way to get in a relaxed state and think about the things that are making you happy.

4. Sitting Position You can sit up after a few minutes and take the time to repeat the process once again if you want something more challenging or if you feel like being active.

5. Balancing Pose The next step is to stand up while you are holding a balancing pose for at least 3 minutes. You can do the tree pose, half moon, or warrior 1 pose to get in better shape and have a stronger core. You will feel much more flexible when you are done with this exercise and you should focus on getting a good stretch in your legs and back.

6. Standing Position Next, you should stand up while focusing on moving your body for another 2 minutes. While holding this position, you want to move around as much as possible so that you start burning fat from different areas of your body.

Conclusion

There are so many great exercises that you can do when working out in a group that can have an amazing impact on your life. You should definitely try these out because they are all exercises that someone else has already done and loved. If you want to get the best results possible, then focus on eating a healthy diet and exercising consistently. If you want extra motivation, then join a group and get better goals with friends! It's important for everyone to move their body and create new habits every day so that they can get healthier over time.

There are so many fun and interesting exercises that you can do when working out in a group, so it's important for everyone to try these out today. Who knows, you might even get the best results possible because of the people around you! It is also important to practice deep breathing every day for a few minutes so that you can calm down and relax your body when you are feeling anxious. This might be the most crucial part of working out in a group because it will get easier as time goes on. If you start focusing on your breathing every day, then it will only get easier for everyone who is living life with anxiety.

The 15-Day Women's Health Book of 15-Minute Workouts

The Time-Saving Program to Raise a Leaner, Stronger, More Muscular You

Anphora Cooper

Table of Contents

Introduction

The 15-Day Fast Track to the Core Program is exactly that...a program that walks you step by step through a 15-minute workout template designed to take your body from a fat-storing machine into a lean, mean, calorie burning machine. OK, so you don't burn calories while sleeping or when you're sitting at your desk, but when you are exercising vigorously like in the 15-Minute Workout, you torch calories and fat at an accelerated rate. The program is designed to get the most out of each workout session by working every muscle group with tri-sets and supersets. The tri-sets and supersets are done so that you are constantly changing the angle of your muscles and joints. This keeps the workout from getting tedious and monotonous. It also increases your metabolism, thus preventing you from getting bored with the workouts.

This program is also designed to be as easy as possible in regard to equipment. I have tried my best to build a program that requires no equipment at all, or if you do have equipment, it should be simple and easy to get your hands on if you don't already own it. The only equipment you need is a set of dumbbells, though I do highly suggest you use a core stabilization ball and a resistance band. You can go to any department store and pick up these items, or if you are like me, your local grocery store has these readily available. The way I look at it is that if they sell it in the grocery store, then it must be pretty good for me! Now before we get into the program itself, I want to give you some tips on what to do with your day between workout sessions. We're not going to make our workouts longer but we will make them more productive by adding just two minutes of cardio work between the warm-up and cool-down period. This will help you burn more fat and calories throughout the day in between your workout sessions. How do I know what to do? Well, a lot of the things I have learned about working out is by studying bodybuilders. Bodybuilders aren't just people who want to be big and bulky...they also must have an incredible degree of muscular definition. The reason for this is that they are judged by how ripped their muscles are as well as how big they are when it comes to competitions such as the Mr. and Miss shows or Mr. Olympia! Bodybuilders know that if you wanted to win, you needed every muscle fibre in your body working together and functioning at its maximum capacity all the time. The only way you can do this is by having some sort of cardiovascular training done daily.

Chapter 1: What is the 15-Minute workouts?

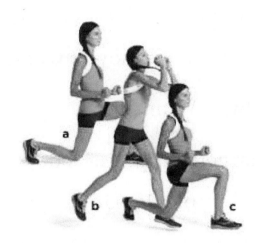

Work Smarter, Not Harder

Every second counts during your busy day—which is why you need a workout program that doesn't take up any of your precious minutes. So we asked our Men's Health Personal Trainer of the Year, Rachel Cosgrove, co-owner of Results Fitness in California and one of the country's top trainers, to create a fast workout routine for women. This 15-day plan will get you looking and feeling better fast.

Each day's workout targets a specific body part and burns about 400 calories. That's an extra 400 calories burned each day, just like that. And, since you're only doing 15 minutes at a time, you can squeeze in these workouts anytime—no excuses! This plan is designed to be easy to follow at home or at the gym. You'll do seven supersets—a superset is when you alternate one set of an exercise with one set of another, back and forth without resting in between. The only rest you get is when it says REST (about a minute). Cosgrove will show you how it works in the video above.

Targeted Training for Busy Women

Each day's workout targets a specific body part with the goal of burning 400 calories. Example: If you do the plan on Monday and Wednesday, your week will be broken down as such: Monday—legs day and upper back day; Wednesday—arms and abs. This allows you to target your hard-to-tone trouble spots in just 15 minutes a day! The workouts are designed to be performed at home or at the gym. You'll do seven supersets—a superset is when you alternate one set of an exercise with one set of another, back and forth without resting in between.

A Healthier Lifestyle

Adding more exercise to your life can only benefit you, provided you exercise safely as discussed in more detail in the next chapter. However, if you are working out to lose weight in addition to becoming more physically fit, you will need to make changes to your diet as well.

The 15-Minute Body Fix will work best when accompanied by these changes. Observing portion sizes, choosing foods that are more nutritious, and limiting sugar, starch and alcohol will improve your health and the effectiveness of your workout.

Be aware, it's not necessary to change radically all aspects of your life at once. In fact, this can sabotage your plans before you really get started by overwhelming your system. Add elements of the 15-Minute Body Fix gradually to your life, and continue adding consistently until you are meeting your final goal.

All You Need Is You

A common complaint about beginning a fitness routine is expense: extensive equipment and videos to buy, or a pricey gym membership. All the workouts in the 15-Minute Body Fix are specifically chose to require little more equipment than your body weight.

Body weight workouts are designed to use your own weight instead of a dumbbell. These kinds of exercises place your body in what is called a disadvantaged position, requiring more strength to make the move. Pushups are the most famous of these exercises, but there are many more. These workouts also usually require the use of several muscle groups, so even if they are zone targeted, you will still continue to strengthen your other parts.

If any other equipment is involved, it will be a common household item, like a towel or a chair. You may also need to use a wall stabilize yourself. You will need a timer. However, a common kitchen timer will do, as will the stopwatch function on most cell phones. No fancy fitness equipment is needed for the 15-Minute Body Fix.

Chapter 2: The Science of Leanness

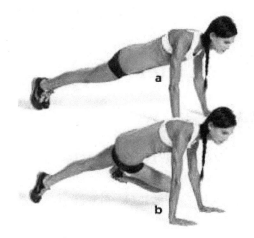

This is the most important chapter in the book. This chapter will teach you everything you need to know about how the human body burns fat and how you can rev up your metabolism so it's operating at its maximum efficiency even if you're not working out. I will also be covering a condition called insulin resistance which is a condition that slows down your metabolism and makes it harder for your body to burn fat. The good news is that insulin resistance is preventable by making small changes in everyday life. It's not something you just have to live with. You will find that in this program, the majority of your workouts focus around the muscles in the core area. The reason for this is because the core is considered to be one of the most important areas for increasing calorie burning. I will also be teaching you how to rev up your metabolism with some simple but very effective exercises. To top it off, I'm also going to teach you about what and when to eat so that you can get all of the fat-burning benefits possible out of your diet plan!

Leanness Is NOT a Four-Letter Word

We have to change the way we look at fat and leanness in the modern day. The fitness world has made us think that being "fat" is something to be ashamed of and that putting on lean muscle is something that you have to work forever for. I'm here to tell you that this is simply not true! It's not true because all of us have fat on our bodies. We need fat to survive! It is true that our bodies can become much healthier if we have more lean muscle on our bodies and less fat but that's not the key. The key is getting leaner while preserving as much muscle tissue as possible. There are some people out there who believe that it's easier to lose weight by burning off as much of the muscle tissue as possible while you're going on a diet. The reason some people think this way is because they are always hungry and they feel lethargic. This is a complete lie! The easiest way to lose weight and keep your muscles intact is to consume just enough nutrients so you don't lose any muscle mass while losing body fat. If you consume an extreme amount of lean protein and just the right amount of carbohydrates, your body will enter a state called ketosis which is a state in which your body burns fat for energy instead of carbohydrates. The only time that carbs are burned is during intense exercise like sprinting. This mean that if you're at a standstill, your body is going to burn fat for energy instead of carbs. Keep in mind that this approach to getting leaner has to be done with long-term consistency. You cannot do this program once every two months and expect to see good results. You can only get the good results by making small changes to your daily life and doing it consistently over time. The worst thing that you can do is to try this program for 3 days and then quit. If you do that, all the time and money that you spent on your supplements will have been a waste. Over the next few sections, I'm going to teach you everything that I have learned over the past 12 years about losing fat while keeping muscle.

Diet

I would like to say it straight out the gate…"There is no quick fix diet!" There are some people who may lose fat quickly but those people are not eating healthy either. Just because you aren't hungry doesn't mean it isn't hurting your body. You will not get the best results with those crazy 3 day diets that you see on TV. Also, if there was a quick fix to losing fat, I could be gone by now. I would have already made my millions and wouldn't be writing these messages to you. There is no magic diet pill or potion that will make it easy for you to lose fat. The old adage "you can't out train a bad diet" cannot be put any more accurately than it is in this sentence. A good diet plays a significant role in getting leaner or building muscle because it is used as the source for your energy (calories) for your body to burn off of. If you don't have the proper nutrients coming in from your diet, your body is going to be forced to tap into muscles and fat tissue for energy. So having a good diet is a must for everyone, no matter what his or her goals may be.

Dieting Tips

1) Cut your portions- The easiest way to start decreasing the amount of calories that you are taking in is to simply cut your portion sizes down. Most people tend to eat overly large portions that main reason being that people cannot deal with having food go away on their plates. If you take in a large portion and finish it all, you feel accomplished. If the food that you ate was low calorie, then there shouldn't be anything to feel accomplished about. So I suggest taking your regular plate of food and half the size so that you're consuming less calories at each sitting. After the first week or two, get another plate of half the size and half with your original sized plate which will now be your medium sized plate. This will help

you get into a routine of eating smaller portions by simply changing out your plates.

2) Eat more often- With the first tip, we want to start becoming in tune with our body's natural hunger signals. We can do this by simply eating more often. I suggest eating 4 meals a day, and 2 snacks. How you eat is not important as long as you are eating smaller portions and getting enough nutrients each day. As I will discuss in my nutrition plan, your meals should consist of a lean protein, fibre filled carbohydrate and a low glycemic index (low sugar) carbohydrate. This is just the basic outline for eating. As we get into the plan in the next few sections, I am going to tell you exactly what to eat for each meal.

3) Avoid sweeteners- Many people turn to sweeteners in order to cut calories from their diet and still have dessert. These sweeteners are usually found in desserts and beverages like soda or juice with little or no real nutritional value. These types of foods will sabotage your efforts because you will simply fill up on them while not getting enough nutrients in your body. The best thing to do is avoid these types of foods all together. This may sound like it's impossible but if you just put in a little extra effort into planning your meals ahead of time, you will find that it's really not that hard and you

will actually be able to enjoy more variety in your diet. I'm not suggesting that you have to cut out desserts for the rest of your life but what I am saying is that if you are trying to get leaner, then it doesn't make any sense at all to eat something that is going to sabotage your efforts.

4) Avoid Sodium- You may have heard this before...but sodium makes us retain water. If you are retaining water, it makes it look like you're not losing fat because your muscles are not as defined as they could be. So this is another area where you need to cut corners. Salt your food sparingly and find a low sodium sports drink or water if you are out and about. If you don't have time to prepare your own meals, try finding restaurants that serve mainly seafood or eat at home. It's much easier for them to control their sodium levels than other types of restaurants.

5) Take your vitamins- Many times, when people go on a diet, they tend to forget about their vitamins and multivitamins. You should always take them even if you are eating a healthy diet. Vitamins and minerals are what make up muscles so without them, you will be losing weight from your muscles instead of fat. A fat loss and muscle building supplement is also a good option for you to use if

you just aren't getting enough nutrients in your body each day (I will discuss this in my nutrition plan).

6) Keep Hydrated- I'm sure you've heard this many times but it's important so I'll say it again...Keep Hydrated! You should shoot for at least 8 glasses of water a day. Most people get all of their water from drinks like soda or juice which are just sugar water with no nutritional value what so ever.

7) Get Enough Sleep- I have already discussed how important sleep is in making muscle gains but another big reason why it's important is because your metabolism is highest when you're sleeping. This means that you should be getting enough sleep each night. If you're only sleeping 5 hours per night, then try to get more by either going to bed earlier or waking up later in the morning.

Chapter 3: How to Maximize Post-Workout Recovery so You Can Train Harder and Recover Faster.

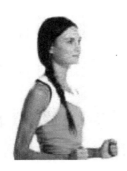

If you want to build a lean and muscular body, you have to train hard and often. Training hard is one thing if you can recover quickly, but if your muscles have a difficult time recovering after a heavy weight training session then all your hard work will be for nothing.

The goal of this chapter is to show you exactly what foods and supplements you can use to help your body recover fast from exercise.

1) Eat smart before going to bed- Try eating more the night before so that you wake up with an empty stomach (don't eat within 3 hours of going to sleep). Make sure your last meal before bed consists of mostly protein. This will help your body repair and recover from weight training while you sleep.

2) Sleep long enough- Not getting enough sleep is the main reason why people can't recover from exercise, because you body needs rest and recuperation. The average person should get between 7-9 hours of sleep per night.

3) Eat protein every 3-4 hours while awake- If you wake up at 6am, try eating a snack that consists of protein like a piece or two of chicken or drink whey protein (depending on your schedule). Then, eat a main meal that consists of a protein source like steak or chicken with a carbohydrate source. Then, have another snack that consists of protein like whey protein or a piece of deli turkey an hour or so after you eat your meal. Then, have another meal an hour after you have your snack and then eat dinner quite late at night (this way you will wake up with an empty stomach). Also, make sure to drink plenty of water to stay hydrated. If you are unable to eat every 3-4 hours while awake then take some type of protein supplement that uses slow-digesting proteins for long lasting amino acid delivery (whey is fast-digesting, casein is slow-digesting).

4) Take supplements- I would recommend taking some type of protein supplement before, during, and after exercise. You can use whey protein, casein protein, milk proteins (such as Optimum

Nutrition 100% Whey Gold Standard), etc. I would also recommend using a multivitamin every day as well as 6-8 grams of BCAA's before and after exercise (I take Optimum Nutrition Amino Energy due to the fact that it contains creatine monohydrate). I recommend using creatine monohydrate because it has been proven to increase strength and lean muscle tissue over a period of time when taken consistently.

5) Eat regularly- Eating many small meals throughout the day is better for recovery than eating a few big meals.

6) Eat more fruits and vegetables- Fruits and vegetables contain important micronutrients that are important for recovery. Also, fruits and vegetables contain carbohydrates which you can absorb quickly to replenish muscle glycogen stores.

7) Eat healthy fats- Healthy fats such as olive oil, coconut oil, flaxseed oil, avocados, nuts, etc. help your body absorb the fat soluble vitamins A,D, E and K from the foods you eat.

8) Drink milk- Milk contains both slow-digesting proteins (casein) and fast-digesting proteins (whey). This makes milk a great post workout supplement.

9) Drink alcohol moderately- Drinking a glass of red wine daily has been shown to improve recovery from exercise.

10) Drink coffee- Research has shown that the amino acid L-Carnitine is found in higher levels in people who drink coffee compared to people who don't drink it. This is important because L-Carnitine helps transport fatty acids into the mitochondria of muscle cells so that they can be used as fuel for energy. The more fatty acids you can get into your mitochondria, the more fat you will burn throughout the day. Also, caffeine in coffee stimulates your central nervous system to make it easy for you to wake up and become highly alert.

Maximizing Post-Workout Recovery

Here is the list of foods and supplements that will help maximize post workout recovery:

1. Lean meats like chicken, turkey, and beef as well as fish

2. Eggs

3. Plant based protein powders

4. Whole milk

5. Whey protein powders (fast absorbing)

6. Casein protein powders (slow absorbing)

7. Multivitamins- Look for ones that contain calcium, magnesium, zinc, B vitamins, vitamin D3 (cholecalciferol), etc…

8. BCAA supplements- Drink these before and after training.

9. Creatine monohydrate

10. Caffeine from coffee or green tea

11. Fruits and vegetables

12. Healthy fats like olive oil, avocados, nuts, fatty fish (e.g., salmon), etc...

13. Milk- Consume this right after you train because it has both fast-digesting whey protein as well as slow-digesting casein protein in it (whey is fast digesting; casein is slow digesting).

14. Alcohol in moderation (e.g., 1 glass of red wine a day) has been shown to improve recovery from exercise .

Chapter 4: The Science of Muscular Strength

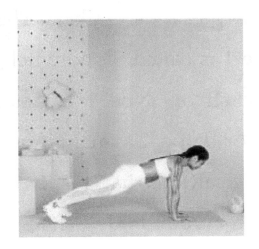

This chapter will teach you everything you need to know about building muscle. I'm not going to be teaching you how to do hundreds of different exercises. Instead, I'm going to be teaching you the most effective compound exercises (multi-joint) for each body part in terms of developing overall strength and increasing lean muscle mass. You will notice that there is a lot of attention paid towards your core muscles. Your core muscles are considered to be the most important muscle group in your body because they play a significant role in stabilizing your spine and increasing calorie burning. I will also be teaching you the different types of muscle fibres and how they help your body in everyday activities. Understanding how muscles work will help you to know what you need to do in order to build strength and muscle.

Muscular Strength and Development Facts

1) There are 2 types of muscle fibres found in our bodies. These are known as Type 1 and Type 2 muscle fibres. There is a simple way to remember them...Type 1 is called Slow twitch and Type 2 is called Fast Twitch. Slow twitch or Type 1 is designed for endurance, whereas fast Twitch or Type 2's main function is power. Slow twitch fibres burn more calories than fast twitch fibres which make them the best choice for your body when it comes to losing fat while preserving as much muscle as possible.

2) In order to build strength and aesthetics, you need to focus on compound exercises that work the major muscle groups of your body. Compound exercises are multijoint exercises (exercises that involve more than one major body part) that use large, powerful movements in order to help your body develop overall strength. These are going to be the exercises that I will be focusing on for you over the next few chapters.

3) Whenever you feel fatigued during an exercise, it is usually a sign that you should stop the exercise and not push through with prolonged muscle failure. Prolonged muscle failure can cause your muscles to have delayed onset muscle soreness (DOMS) as well as take longer for your muscles to repair and rebuild themselves.

4) In order to build strength and muscle, you must eat enough calories and protein. Calories are the basic building blocks of energy needed for your muscles to repair themselves after an intense workout. Protein not only builds your muscles but it also helps them retain water which gives you a pumped look. I will discuss all of these nutrients as we get into my nutrition plan later on in this book.

5) Although I said that slow twitch fibres are more efficient for burning calories, they do not have the ability to explode or generate as much power as fast twitch fibres can. This is why you need to use both types of exercises in order to develop strength and aesthetics (looks).

How The Body Creates Muscle

The task of strength and muscle development can be very complicated. I'm not going to get into the details of it, but I will give you a brief overview of what is happening during a typical muscle building process.

As we begin to lift heavy weights, two important reactions take place in the body. The first is that the brain releases a chemical known as adrenaline (epinephrine). Adrenaline speeds up the heart rate and makes more blood available for muscular contraction. This reaction increases muscular strength which is needed as your body begins to lift heavier weights. This reaction occurs for only a short period of time in order to maximize your ability to lift while not overworking your body.

The second reaction, which can last up to 48 hours after a rigorous workout session, is when your body releases growth hormone (GH). During this time, GH stimulates the muscles to repair themselves as quickly as possible. This allows your body to build more muscle for future workouts. GH is also responsible for the burning sensation you feel 24-48 hours later.

In order to develop strength and increase lean muscle mass, you need to keep challenging your body by upping the intensity of your workouts. Your body will adapt within 3-4 weeks if you are training properly and doing more than just lifting light weights with poor form. You must keep your brain thinking that you're not capable of handling the amount of weight you are lifting if you want to continue to make progress.

Chapter 5: How to Build Lean Muscle (and Raise Your Metabolism)

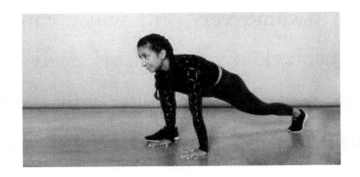

This chapter will be all about developing lean muscle mass. I will be discussing the six steps to building muscle and the type of equipment you should be using for each step. I will also give you a sample workout schedule to follow at the end. The first step to building muscle is stretching which I will discuss in this chapter as well.

I'm going to start by talking about how important it is for your muscles to stretch before and after every workout you do (this includes stretching your core). The main reason why it's important is because if you stretch the muscles, tendons and ligaments before a workout, then they are much more apt to being stretched during the workout as well. If you stretch before a workout, then your body will be much more flexible and better capable of handling the stress of your weight training. Lifting weights puts a lot of pressure on the muscles that you are exercising. If you don't stretch before your workout, then the pressure on those muscles can cause them to tighten up and become very stiff which can result in muscle strains. I'm sure you know what this feels like from either experience or just seeing someone else with a muscle pull while working out. This is also known as delayed onset muscle soreness (DOMS) which I will discuss later on.

Understand that all of your workouts should be done in a progressive manner which means that each workout gets more intense than the last and that the weight you are using increases every week. There are six steps to developing lean muscle mass. These steps include: stretching, dynamic flexibility, active flexibility, traditional strength training, pre-exhaustion and super sets. Here they are in more detail:

1) Stretching- Before doing any kind of weight training or flexibility exercises, you need to stretch for at least 10 minutes or until you feel completely stretched out. When doing this stretch routine, make sure to hold each stretch for 15 seconds before moving on to the next one (I'll discuss how to do each stretch later).

Stretching will do two things for you. First of all, it will improve your flexibility which is needed in order to perform some of the exercises I'll be teaching you. Secondly, it will help to keep your muscles from becoming tight which can result from being under too much stress while weight training (I explained how this works in the "Building Lean Mass" chapter).

2) Dynamic Flexibility- Dynamic flexibility is very similar to static stretching except that dynamic flexibility incorporates movement into the stretch so that you are actually moving through your range of motion. This type of stretching should also be done before your weight training workouts as well. The best way to do this is to start by loosening up your muscles and then move through your range of motion as you would when doing the actual exercise. I'll demonstrate this in more detail later on.

3) Active Flexibility- Active flexibility is basically doing the opposite of static stretching. Instead of holding a stretch for 15 seconds, you're going to hold it for 15 seconds or however long you can before your muscles begin to tighten back up and then contract yourself for 15 seconds (this applies when doing crunches or sit ups). This type of stretching should also be done before each workout session, especially lower body days.

4) Traditional Strength Training- This is what most people think of when they hear the words "weight training". This is where you use

heavy weights and perform an exercise in a controlled manner in order to develop the strength of that particular muscle. You should use between 3-5 sets per exercise and do 4-6 repetitions for each set. When you are doing these exercises, don't just lift the weight up and down without any control. You should be using your muscles to move the weight up and down. If you are just moving sluggishly through your range of motion then it means that you aren't getting a good workout.

5) Pre-Exhaust Training- Here you will be doing a set of an exercise for one particular muscle group and then immediately (with no rest in between) doing a set of an exercise that works the same muscle group but with a different range of motion. This is considered to be one superset. This is another way to challenge your body so that it continually adapts to the stress you are putting on it.

6) Super Sets- Here you will be doing two exercises for the same muscle group without any rest in between them. You should do each super set for 3 sets per exercise and 6 repetitions per set (I'll explain how to choose the right amount weight later).

Sample Workout Schedule

I am going to give you a sample workout schedule that you can try. This is a six day per week split routine and will involve several strength training exercises as well as active flexibility, dynamic flexibility and stretching for each muscle group. The first four days will be for training your upper body and the last two days will be for your lower body. It's important that you change up the order of these workouts every other week at least so that your body doesn't adapt to the workout routine repetition. Before each workout, warm up for 10-15 minutes by either doing some cardio or jogging in place (I will discuss warming up in more detail later on).

This schedule should be used as an example for you to follow and not as a "set in stone" plan. You need to change it up each time to make sure your body doesn't adapt to the same workout routine.

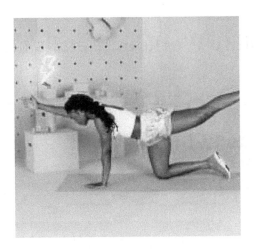

Day 1: Chest/Triceps (Rest Day)

A. Barbell Bench Press 3 x 8-12 reps

B. Cable Crossover 2 x 15-20 reps

C. Chest Stretch 5-10 reps (hold for 15 seconds)

D. Triceps Stretch (active flexibility) 5-10 reps (hold for 15 seconds)

E. Triceps Stretch (static flexibility) 10-15 reps

F. Clasping Triceps Stretch 10-15 reps

G. Clasping Rear Delt Stretch 10-15 reps

H. Chest Stretch 5-10 reps (hold for 15 seconds)

I. Triceps Stretch (active flexibility) 5-10 reps (hold for 15 seconds)

J. Triceps Stretch (static flexibility) 10-15 reps

K. Clasping Triceps Stretch 10-15 reps

L. Clasping Rear Delt Stretch 5-10 reps

M. Active Back Flexibility Workout (details later)

Day 2: Back/Biceps (Rest Day)

A. Barbell Deadlift 3 x 8-12 reps

B. Seated Row 3 x 8-12 reps

C. Lat Stretch 5-10 reps (hold for 15 seconds)

D. Bicep Stretch (active flexibility) 5-10 reps (hold for 15 seconds)

E. Bicep Stretch (static flexibility) 10-15 reps

F. Kneeling Overhead Triceps Stretch 10-15 reps

G. Head to Toe Bicep Stretch 10-15 reps

H. Lat Stretch 5-10 reps (hold for 15 seconds)

I. Bicep Stretch (active flexibility) 5-10 reps (hold for 15 seconds)

J. Bicep Stretch (static flexibility) 10-15 reps

K. Kneeling Overhead Triceps Stretch 10-15 reps

L. Head to Toe Bicep Stretch 10-15 reps

M. Lat Stretch 5-10 reps (hold for 15 seconds)

N. Bicep Stretch (active flexibility) 5-10 reps (hold for 15 seconds)

O. Bicep Stretch (static flexibility) 10-15 reps

P. Kneeling Overhead Triceps Stretch 10-15 reps

Q. Head to Toe Bicep Stretch 10-15 reps

Day 3: Legs/Core(Rest Day)

A. Barbell Deadlift 3 x 8-12 reps

B. Leg Press 3 x 8-12 reps

C. Cable Woodchop 2 x 15-20 reps

D. Hip Flexor Stretch 5-10 reps (hold for 15 seconds; each leg)

E. Hamstring Stretch (active flexibility) 5-10 reps (hold for 15 seconds; each leg)

F. Hamstring Stretch (static flexibility) 10-15 reps

G. Quad Stretch 5-10 reps (hold for 15 seconds; each leg)

H. Lat Stretch 5-10 reps (hold for 15 seconds; each leg)

I. Bicep Stretch (active flexibility) 5-10 reps (hold for 15 seconds; each arm)

J. Bicep Stretch (static flexibility) 10-15 reps

K. Kneeling Overhead Triceps Stretch 10-15 reps

L. Clasping Triceps Stretch 10-15 reps

M. Clasping Rear Delt Stretch 5-10 reps

N. Core Flexibility Workout (details later)

Day 4: Chest/Triceps (Rest Day)

A. Flat Barbell Bench Press 3 x 8-12 reps

B. Decline Push Up 2 x 15-20 reps

C. Chest Stretch 5-10 reps (hold for 15 seconds)

D. Tricep Stretch (active flexibility) 5-10 reps (hold for 15 seconds)

E. Tricep Stretch (static flexibility) 10-15 reps

F. Clasping Tricep Stretch 10-15 reps

G. Clasping Rear Delt Stretch 10-15 reps

H. Chest Stretch 5-10 reps (hold for 15 seconds)

I. Tricep Stretch (active flexibility) 5-10 reps (hold for 15 seconds)

J. Tricep Stretch (static flexibility) 10-15 reps

K. Clasping Tricep Stretch 10-15 reps

L. Clasping Rear Delt Stretch 5-10 reps

M. Active Back Flexibility Workout (details later)

Day 5: Back/Biceps (Rest Day)

A. Good Morning 3 x 8-12 reps

B. Deadlift 3 x 8-12 reps

C. Lat Stretch 5-10 reps (hold for 15 seconds; each arm)

D. Bicep Stretch (active flexibility) 5-10 reps (hold for 15 seconds; each arm)

E. Bicep Stretch (static flexibility) 10-15 reps

F. Kneeling Overhead Tricep Stretch 10-15 reps

G. Clasping Front Delt Stretch 10-15 reps

H. Lat Stretch 5-10 reps (hold for 15 seconds; each arm)

I. Bicep Stretch (active flexibility) 5-10 reps (hold for 15 seconds; each arm)

J. Bicep Stretch (static flexibility) 10-15 reps

K. Kneeling Overhead Tricep Stretch 10-15 reps

L. Clasping Front Delt Stretch 5-10 reps

M. Lat Stretch 5-10 reps (hold for 15 seconds; each arm)

N. Bicep Stretch (active flexibility) 5-10 reps (hold for 15 seconds; each arm)

O. Bicep Stretch (static flexibility) 10-15 reps

P. Kneeling Overhead Tricep Stretch 10-15 reps

Q. Clasping Front Delt Stretch 5-10 reps

R. Lat Stretch 5-10 reps (hold for 15 seconds; each arm)

S. Bicep Stretch (active flexibility) 5-10 reps (hold for 15 seconds; each arm)

T. Bicep Stretch (static flexibility) 10-15 reps

U. Kneeling Overhead Tricep Stretch 10-15 reps

V. Clasping Front Delt Stretch 5-10 reps

W. Lat Stretch 5-10 reps (hold for 15 seconds; each arm)

X. Bicep Stretch (active flexibility) 5-10 reps (hold for 15 seconds; each arm)

Y. Bicep Stretch (static flexibility) 10-15 reps

Z. Kneeling Overhead Tricep Stretch 10-15 reps

AA. Clasping Front Delt Stretch 5-10 reps

BB. Lat Stretch 5-10 reps (hold for 15 seconds; each arm)

CC. Bicep Stretch (active flexibility) 5-10 reps (hold for 15 seconds; each arm)

DD. Bicep Stretch (static flexibility) 10-15 reps

EE. Kneeling Overhead Tricep Stretch 10-15 reps

FF. Clasping Front Delt Stretch 5-10 reps

GG. Lat Stretch 5-10 reps (hold for 15 seconds; each arm)

HH. Bicep Stretch (active flexibility) 5-10 reps (hold for 15 seconds; each arm)

II. Bicep Stretch (static flexibility) 10-15 reps

JJ. Kneeling Overhead Tricep Stretch 10-15 reps

KK. Clasping Front Delt Stretch 5-10 reps

LL. Lat Stretch 5-10 reps (hold for 15 seconds; each arm)

MM. Bicep Stretch (active flexibility) 5-10 reps (hold for 15 seconds; each arm)

Chapter 6: Resize Your Thighs

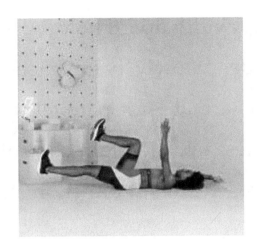

These workouts will focus on your thighs and legs. Although your Full Body Workouts work these muscles, if this is a trouble spot for you in terms of strength, you may want a more targeted routine.

Leg and Thigh Workout 1

This workout is structured as others you have done, organized into Part A and Part B. You will be learning some new exercises, and using some you have already learned.

Part A

Do 10 Squat Jumps are performed safely this way:

Stand with feet together and hands on hips. Keeping your back straight, slowly bend your knees until they are at a 90 degree angle, then thrust upwards, jumping as high as you can. When you land, bring your knees back up to a 90-degree angle. This is one rep.

1. Squats

Stand tall with feet hip-width apart, holding a set of 5- to 15-pound dumbbells at your sides. Slowly bend knees and hips and lower your body until thighs are at least parallel to the floor. Keep head facing forward and chest up. Maintain control of the weights at all times during exercise. Reverse direction to return to starting position and repeat for reps.

2. Lunges

Holding 5- to 15-pound dumbbells in each hand, step forward with left foot and lower body into a lunge until front thigh is parallel to floor; keep back leg straight so that knee does not extend past toe as you go down. Return to start and repeat with right leg. That's 1 rep.

3. Triceps Extensions

Grasp a pair of dumbbells and stand with knees bent and weights hanging at your sides. Straighten arms in front of you until they form a 90-degree angle with your upper arms; keep elbows pointing down toward the floor throughout exercise. Press weights overhead until arms are straight but not locked, then bend elbows to lower them back down. That's 1 rep.

4. Pushups

Start in an elevated pushup position, with hands on the floor directly beneath shoulders, body straight from head to heels, legs extended behind you and toes pointing forward (A). Bend elbows to lower body until chest nearly touches floor (B). Push back up to start and repeat for reps.

5. Squats Alternate with Biceps Curls

Hold a pair of dumbbells in each hand, arms hanging at your sides. Keeping back straight, bend knees and hips as if you were sitting into a chair (A) until thighs are at least parallel to the floor. Now stand and push weights toward ceiling until elbows are fully extended (B). Reverse movement to return to start and repeat for reps.

Do 10 Side Lunges.

Complete Part A 8 times.

Rest 2 minutes.

Part B

Do 10 Jumping Lunges.

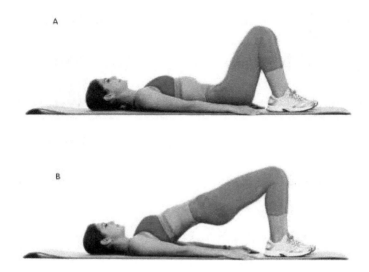

Do 10 Glute Bridges. This is how to do **Glute Bridges:**

1. Lie in neutral position on your back on the floor. A neutral position is not totally flat, nor totally arched. You should be able to slip you hand part way into the curve of your back, but it should not fit all the way.

2. Place your feet, at hip width, evenly on the floor, with your toes pointing forward and your knees bent.

3. Contract your abdominal muscles. Imagine your belly button pulling in toward your spine. Keep your muscles this way throughout the exercise.

4. Push your hips up through your heels. You back should remain in the neutral position. If you back begins to arch or you feel pressure on your neck, you have done too fat.

5. You will keep your abdominals contracted as you lower your hips to the floor.

6. You should not truly rest in between repetitions, only lightly touch the floor.

Complete Part B 8 times.

Rest 2 minutes.

Continue cycling through Parts A and B for 15 minutes.

Leg and Thigh Workout 2

This workout is organized as a circuit. This means that you go from one exercise to another with only a 10 second rest in between. You are measuring by time instead of repetitions, so do each move as quickly and correctly as you can.

Do Squats for 30 seconds

Rest for 10 seconds.

Do Single-Leg Deadlifts for 30 seconds. The **Single-Leg Deadlift** is performed properly this way:

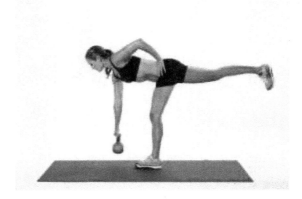

1. Begin in a standing position.

2. Raise one leg straight behind you with your toes pointing downwards.

3. As you raise your leg, bend forward from the hips, keeping your back flat. Keep your neck aligned with your spine, and loose, not tensed.

4. Your hands will be perpendicular to your chest. Do not reach towards the floor, as this may cause you to round your back.

5. Bend only as far as flexibility will allow, while keeping your core tight and your back straight.

6. Continue with your abs tight and your back straight as you lower your leg and return to a standing position.

7. Do not alternate legs until the next circuit. Stick with the single leg.

Rest 10 seconds.

Do Glute Bridges for 30 seconds.

Rest for 1 minute.

Repeat circuit for the entire 15 minutes. If you can only do a few exercises in the 30 seconds, do not get discouraged. You will get faster.

Lower Body Workout 3

This workout follows the pattern, which should now be familiar to you, of 10 repetitions and Jumping Jacks in between.

Begin with 10 Reverse Lunges.

Then do Jumping Jacks until your timer says 1 minute has passed.

At minute 1, do 10 Side Lunges.

Do Jumping Jacks until minute 2.

At minute 2, Do 10 Squats.

Do Jumping Jacks until minute 3.

At minute 3, do 10 Single-Leg Deadlifts.

Do Jumping Jacks until minute 4.

At minute 4, start again.

Do not forget to switch legs on your Single-Leg Deadlifts when you get there.

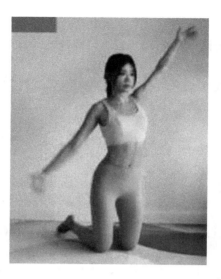

Leg and Thigh Workout 4

This workout will follow the established pattern with Part A and Part B.

Part A

1. Do 10 Jumping Lunges.

2. Rest 10 seconds.

3. Do 10 Single-Leg Deadlifts.

4. Rest 10 seconds.

5. Repeat Part A 8 times.

Part B

1. Do 10 Glute Bridges.

2. Rest 10 seconds.

3. Do 10 Squats.

4. Rest 10 seconds.

5. Repeat Part B 8 times.

6. Cycle between Parts A for the remainder of 15 minutes.

Leg and Thigh Workout 5

This workout is organized as a circuit.

1. Begin with 30 seconds of Jumping Lunges.

2. Rest 10 seconds.

3. Then, do 30 second of Reverse Lunges.

4. Rest 10 seconds.

5. Next, do 30 seconds of Squat Jumps.

6. Rest 1 minute.

Repeat this circuit as many times as you can in 15 minutes.

Chapter 7: The Lean 15-Minute Workouts for Building Muscle and Losing Fat

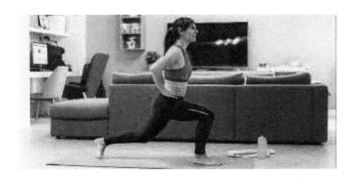

When it comes to building muscle, the biggest obstacle that women face is finding the time to work out. That's why I created The Lean 15 Workouts—the most efficient and effective way for women to burn fat and build lean muscle in only 15 minutes a day. The Lean 15 Workouts take advantage of the body-shaping effects of supersets, which are two exercises performed back-to-back with no rest in between. Supersets force you to work your muscles past their normal failure points, which triggers more growth responses from your body. While you're performing supersets, you'll also be incorporating another muscle-building technique called compound sets, which involve pairing two exercises that work opposing muscle groups. For example, pairing a bench press with a row works your chest and back.

The Lean 15 Workouts employ both of these strategies in dozens of different combinations to help you build and sculpt your entire body. The best part is that each workout keeps your heart rate elevated throughout the entire routine and you only rest when needed—usually between supersets—so you maximize every second of your workout time. The Lean 15 Workouts are divided into two different types of workouts—The Lean 15 Workouts for Beginners and The Lean 15 Workouts for Experienced Exercisers. Below I explain how to use each workout and provide a sample routine that combines exercises from all four phases of the program.

The Lean 15 Workout for Beginners is designed for women who haven't worked out in a while, are new to weight training, or have never lifted weights before. It's also a good option if you've been exercising regularly with moderate intensity but haven't seen any changes in your body or fitness level. The Lean 15 Workout for Beginners will help you build your strength, endurance, and confidence so you can move on to the next phase of the program. The exercises are broken down into four phases—Phase 1: Resistance Training, Phase 2: Strength Training, Phase 3: Advanced Resistance Training and Phase 4: Strength and Power—and each phase works your body in a slightly different way.

In Phase 1: Resistance Training (weeks 1–4), you'll start out with light weights to get used to the exercises and gradually build up your strength. As your muscles get stronger, you'll gradually increase the amount of weight you lift as well as the number of reps you perform. Phase 1: Resistance Training is a great option if you're just starting out with resistance training or you've been working out regularly but haven't seen any changes in your body. Phase 2: Strength Training (weeks 5–8) focuses on increasing the amount of weight you lift for each exercise. To keep your muscles guessing, we incorporate three different supersets — the kickback superset, the press-up superset and the super squat superset — and alternate between them throughout the routine.

The third phase, Phase 3: Advanced Resistance Training (weeks 9–12), builds on the exercises from Phase 2: Strength Training. We also add another superset — this time the single-arm dumbbell row superset — to keep your body working hard. Phase 4: Strength and Power (weeks 13–16) is a repeat of Phase 2: Strength Training. This time, though, you'll be doing many of the exercises for fewer reps and adding more weight to each exercise.

Phases 1: Resistance Training and 2: Strength Training are great options if you've only been exercising for a few weeks or have never lifted weights before. Both phases will help you build strength, endurance and confidence in the gym so you can graduate to the more advanced exercises in Phase 3: Advanced Resistance Training and Phase 4: Strength and Power. The Lean 15 Workout for Experienced Exercisers is designed for women who have been working out regularly with moderate intensity but haven't seen any changes in their body or fitness level. These workouts focus on increasing your weight-training intensity while maintaining the high-energy, fast-paced workouts that I developed for The Lean 15 Workout for Beginners.

For each of the four phases — Phase 1: Resistance Training, Phase 2: Strength Training, Phase 3: Advanced Resistance Training and Phase 4: Strength and Power — you'll perform one set of each exercise in rapid succession with no rest between exercises. Rest only when needed between supersets (usually after you finish a superset). Each phase is slightly different but all four incorporate supersets into the routine. In Phase 1: Resistance Training (weeks 1–4), for example, you'll alternate between two types of supersets — the press-up superset and the kickback superset — and use dumbbells instead of barbells. In Phase 2: Strength Training (weeks 5–8), you'll perform the same exercises as Phase 1: Resistance

Training but this time we'll use barbells and alternate between three different supersets — the press-up superset, the single-arm dumbbell row superset and the super squat superset.

In Phase 3: Advanced Resistance Training (weeks 9–12) you'll do the same exercises from Phase 2 but with a third superset — the cable pulldown superset. In Phase 4: Strength and Power (weeks 13–16), we'll take it up a notch by performing many of the exercises for fewer reps and adding more weight to each exercise.

Phase 1: Resistance Training is a great option if you've only been exercising for a few weeks or if you haven't lifted weights before. This phase will help you build confidence and get comfortable with the exercises. Phase 2: Strength Training is a great option if you've been working out regularly but haven't seen any changes in your body or fitness level. Phase 2 not only helps you build strength but also focuses on increasing endurance by alternating between different supersets and adding variety to the exercises.

Phase 3: Advanced Resistance Training focuses on increasing your weight-training intensity while maintaining the high-energy, fast-paced workouts that worked so well in Phases 1 and 2. Phase 4: Strength and Power is for experienced exercisers who have been working out regularly with moderate intensity but haven't seen the changes in their body or fitness level that they're looking for. This phase helps you build strength and power so you can graduate to the more advanced exercises in Phase 5: Lean 15 Workout to get the lean, toned body you want.

Phase 1: Resistance Training (weeks 1–4) - Alternate between press-up supersets and kickback supersets, using dumbbells instead of barbells.

Phase 2: Strength Training (weeks 5–8) - Alternate between super squat supersets and single-arm dumbbell row supersets, using barbells instead of dumbbells.

Phase 3: Advanced Resistance Training (weeks 9–12) - Alternate between cable pulldown supersets and super squat supersets, using a variety of weight plates attached to one end of the cable.

Phase 4: Strength and Power (weeks 13–16) - Alternate between walking lunges and squat thrusts.

Phase 5: Lean 15 Workout (weeks 17–20) - Alternate between mountain climbers and glute bridges.

Phase 6: Core Challenge Workout (weeks 21–24) - Alternate between Russian twists and crunches with a medicine ball.

Chapter 8: The 15-Day Body of Your Dreams in Just 15 Minutes a Day (or Less)

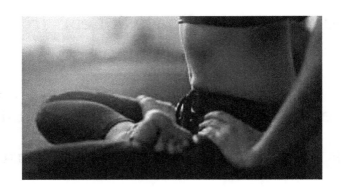

Part I. Introduction to the 15 Day Lean Body Program

The 15 Day Lean Body Program is a variation on the program designed by Martin Rooney and featured in his books. It is ideally suited for those who have a busy schedule but want to stay fit. The 15 Day Lean Body Program uses high intensity interval training (HIIT) to help you build lean muscle mass and burn fat faster than traditional cardio workouts. This quick workout can be done from anywhere with no equipment needed.

The 15 Day Lean Body Program relies on ideal bodyweight exercises to help you build lean muscle mass and burn fat in minimal time. The routines are inspired by the method used by the Australian Army Training Command to train soldiers for fitness and strength, with a specific focus on explosive strength. This method is used by elite athletes around the world.

To get you started, here is a sample routine from the 15 Day Lean Body Program. You can easily follow along with this program in your own home. Feel free to adjust reps or sets, if needed for your fitness level or schedule. Rest as needed between sets and feel free to repeat this workout as many times as you like within a 2-week period. If you need to break up the workout into smaller time periods to accommodate your schedule, that's fine.

• Workout 1 (15 minutes): one set each of squats, lunges, push-ups, and pull-ups

The Bodyweight Cardio Challenge Workout lists the bodyweight cardio exercises that you should use for this 2-week challenge. You will not do burpees because they are a high intensity exercise and therefore you cannot perform them on a day where you will also do bodyweight cardio. Be sure to choose one of the following exercises each time you do bodyweight cardio for the next 14 days.

Workout 2 (15 minutes): Burpee Challenge plus one set of push-ups

The Bodyweight Cardio Challenge Workout lists the bodyweight cardio exercises that you should use for this 2-week challenge. You will not do burpees because they are a high intensity exercise and therefore you cannot perform them on a day where you will also do bodyweight cardio. Be sure to choose one of the following exercises each time you do bodyweight cardio for the next 14 days.

Workout 3 (15 minutes): two sets of each exercise

The Bodyweight Cardio Challenge Workout lists the bodyweight cardio exercises that you should use for this 2-week challenge. You will not do burpees because they are a high intensity exercise and therefore you cannot perform them on a day where you will also do bodyweight cardio. Be sure to choose one of the following exercises each time you do bodyweight cardio for the next 14 days.

Workout 4 (15 minutes): Bear Challenge plus push-ups

The Bodyweight Cardio Challenge Workout lists the bodyweight cardio exercises that you should use for this 2-week challenge. You will not do burpees because they are a high intensity exercise and therefore you cannot perform them on a day where you will also do bodyweight cardio. Be sure to choose one of the following exercises each time you do bodyweight cardio for the next 14 days.

Workout 5 (15 minutes): Mountain Climber Challenge plus pull-ups

The Bodyweight Cardio Challenge Workout lists the bodyweight cardio exercises that you should use for this 2-week challenge. You will not do burpees because they are a high intensity exercise and therefore you cannot perform them on a day where you will also do bodyweight cardio. Be sure to choose one of the following exercises each time you do bodyweight cardio for the next 14 days.

Part II. The Fast Track to the Core Program

The Fast Track to the Core Program uses high intensity interval training (HIIT) to help you build lean muscle mass and burn fat faster than traditional cardio workouts. This 2-week program can be done from anywhere with no equipment needed.

The Fast Track to the Core Programs relies on ideal bodyweight exercises to help you build lean muscle mass and burn fat in minimal time. The routines are inspired by the method used by the Australian Army Training Command to train soldiers for fitness and strength, with a specific focus on explosive strength. This method is used by elite athletes around the world.

To get you started, here is a sample routine from the Fast Track to the Core Program. You can easily follow along with this program in your own home. Feel free to adjust reps or sets, if needed for your fitness level or schedule. Rest as needed between sets and feel free to repeat this workout as many times as you like within a 2-week period. If you need to break up the workout into smaller time periods to accommodate your schedule, that's fine.

• Workout 1 (15 minutes): one set each of squats, lunges, push-ups, and pull-ups

The Bodyweight Cardio Challenge Workout lists the bodyweight cardio exercises that you should use for this 2-week challenge. You will not do burpees because they are a high intensity exercise and therefore you cannot perform them on a day where you will also do bodyweight cardio. Be sure to choose one of the following exercises each time you do bodyweight cardio for the next 14 days.

Workout 2 (15 minutes): Burpee Challenge plus one set of push-ups

The Bodyweight Cardio Challenge Workout lists the bodyweight cardio exercises that you should use for this 2-week challenge. You will not do burpees because they are a high intensity exercise and therefore you cannot perform them on a day where you will also do bodyweight cardio. Be sure to choose one of the following exercises each time you do bodyweight cardio for the next 14 days.

Workout 3 (15 minutes): one set of each exercise

The Bodyweight Cardio Challenge Workout lists the bodyweight cardio exercises that you should use for this 2-week challenge. You will not do burpees because they are a high intensity exercise and therefore you cannot perform them on a day where you will also do bodyweight cardio. Be sure to choose one of the following exercises each time you do bodyweight cardio for the next 14 days.

Workout 4 (15 minutes): Bear Challenge plus push-ups

The Bodyweight Cardio Challenge Workout lists the bodyweight cardio exercises that you should use for this 2-week challenge. You will not do burpees because they are a high intensity exercise and therefore you cannot perform them on a day where you will also do bodyweight cardio. Be sure to choose one of the following exercises each time you do bodyweight cardio for the next 14 days.

Workout 5 (15 minutes): Mountain Climber Challenge plus pull-ups

The Bodyweight Cardio Challenge Workout lists the bodyweight cardio exercises that you should use for this 2-week challenge. You will not do burpees because they are a high intensity exercise and therefore you cannot perform them on a day where you will also do bodyweight cardio. Be sure to choose one of the following exercises each time you do bodyweight cardio for the next 14 days.

Part III. The Fast Track to the Fat Burn Program

The Fast Track to the Fat Burn Program uses high intensity interval training (HIIT) to help you build lean muscle mass and burn fat faster than traditional cardio workouts. This 2-week program can be done from anywhere with no equipment needed."

The Fast Track to the Fat Burn Program relies on ideal bodyweight exercises to help you build lean muscle mass and burn fat in minimal time. The routines are inspired by the method used by the Australian Army Training Command to train soldiers for fitness and strength, with a specific focus on explosive strength. This method is used by elite athletes around the world.

To get you started, here is a sample routine from the Fast Track to the Fat Burn Program. You can easily follow along with this program in your own home. Feel free to adjust reps or sets, if needed for your fitness level or schedule. Rest as needed between sets and feel free to repeat this workout as many times as you like within a 2-week period. If you need to break up the workout into smaller time periods to accommodate your schedule, that's fine.

• Workout 1 (15 minutes): one set each of squats, lunges, push-ups, and pull-ups

The Bodyweight Cardio Challenge Workout lists the bodyweight cardio exercises that you should use for this 2-week challenge. You will not do burpees because they are a high intensity exercise and therefore you cannot perform them on a day where you will also do bodyweight cardio. Be sure to choose one of the following exercises each time you do bodyweight cardio for the next 14 days.

Workout 2 (15 minutes): Burpee Challenge plus one set of push-ups

The Bodyweight Cardio Challenge Workout lists the bodyweight cardio exercises that you should use for this 2-week challenge. You will not do burpees because they are a high intensity exercise and therefore you cannot perform them on a day where you will also do bodyweight cardio. Be sure to choose one of the following exercises each time you do bodyweight cardio for the next 14 days.

Workout 3 (15 minutes): one set of each exercise

The Bodyweight Cardio Challenge Workout lists the bodyweight cardio exercises that you should use for this 2-week challenge. You will not do burpees because they are a high intensity exercise and therefore you cannot perform them on a day where you will also do bodyweight cardio. Be sure to choose one of the following exercises each time you do bodyweight cardio for the next 14 days.

Part IV. Wrapping Up with Fat-Burning Tips from Our All-Star Team

The Fat Burning Plan contains four fat burning workouts to help you create lean muscle mass and burn fat in minimal time. The routines in the program are inspired by the method used by the Australian Army Training Command to train soldiers for fitness and strength, with a specific focus on explosive strength. This method is used by elite athletes around the world.

To get you started, here is a sample routine from the Fat Burning Plan. You can easily follow along with this program in your own home. Feel free to adjust reps or sets, if needed for your fitness level or schedule. Rest as needed between sets and feel free to repeat this workout as many times as you like within a 2-week period. If you need to break up the workout into smaller time periods to accommodate your schedule, that's fine.

• Workout 1 (15 minutes): one set each of squats, lunges, push-ups, and pull-ups

The Bodyweight Cardio Challenge Workout lists the bodyweight cardio exercises that you should use for this 2-week challenge. You will not do burpees because they are a high intensity exercise and therefore you cannot perform them on a day where you will also do bodyweight cardio. Be sure to choose one of the following exercises each time you do bodyweight cardio for the next 14 days.

Workout 2 (15 minutes): Burpee Challenge plus one set of push-ups

The Bodyweight Cardio Challenge Workout lists the bodyweight cardio exercises that you should use for this 2-week challenge. You will not do burpees because they are a high intensity exercise and therefore you cannot perform them on a day where you will also do bodyweight cardio. Be sure to choose one of the following exercises each time you do bodyweight cardio for the next 14 days.

Workout 3 (15 minutes): Bear Challenge plus push-ups

The Bodyweight Cardio Challenge Workout lists the bodyweight cardio exercises that you should use for this 2-week challenge. You will not do burpees because they are a high intensity exercise and therefore you cannot perform them on a day where you will also do bodyweight cardio. Be sure to choose one of the following exercises each time you do bodyweight cardio for the next 14 days.

Workout 4 (15 minutes): Mountain Climber Challenge plus pull-ups

The Bodyweight Cardio Challenge Workout lists the bodyweight cardio exercises that you should use for this 2-week challenge. You will not do burpees because they are a high intensity exercise and therefore you cannot perform them on a day where you will also do bodyweight cardio. Be sure to choose one of the following exercises each time you do bodyweight cardio for the next 14 days.

Chapter 9: Benefits Of 15 Minutes Workout

- One cannot complain that one does not have time to work out, in the busy schedule of life. 15 minutes robust workout technique is commonly being practiced by the working professionals to maintain their work life balance.

- The interval workout with high intensity is said to show better results as compared to normal cardio workout outs which stretch for longer duration.

- The person can decide the kind of work out one wants to plan, to suit his daily needs and his body characteristics.

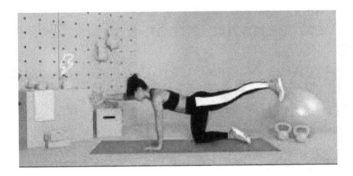

There Are Various Tips Which Needs To Be Followed Before Exercising

1. Start Slow

Any new thing has to be started with lower expectations as it takes time to get used to doing something new and also takes time to get results out of the same. For a start, one should do very basic exercises like running for 10 minutes on a daily basis for next three weeks. Body will need to get used to physical pressure and exercise. If someone starts with a heavy work out then he can seriously damage his internal organs because of excessive heat and sudden increase in body temperature.

2.   Change The Cycle

The exercise should be a onetime permanent set. The exercise should keep changing so that it does not get boring and monotonous. According to the purpose of the exercise one should also change the type and duration of exercise. For example if someone wants to increase the body muscle then he should limit his cardio exercise to a bare minimum and if someone is working out to get lean then his whole workout session should be dedicated to cardio exercises. In cardio exercises also one should take care of alternating the exercise on a daily basis. The person exercising in home can change the options from cycling to rowing to running on a treadmill, for 15 minutes.

3.   Separate Cardio From Strength Training

There are various strength building exercises and many cardio exercises which affects separately to the body. The cardio exercises affect the fat of the body and the strength gaining exercises are specific to body parts. If the person wants to gain strength in his hand or legs then he accordingly does crunches and squats to increasing the leg strength. Now running and cycling also is leg exercise but comes under cardio exercise. It is important to separate the two exercises and do not perform cardio exercise and leg strength increasing exercise in one day. This will lead to fatigue and the purpose of the exercise will not be solved.

4.   Removal Of Fat Burning Zone Myth

Initially it was a common believe that a person need to exercise in 70-80 percent of his maximum heart rate to start the metabolism process and start losing fat. It was also a common believe that one will have to keep working out, in the above mentioned rate, for at least 20 minutes before the fat burning process starts. This, however, has been proven as a myth and now it is accepted that if a person follows interval workout sessions then he can definitely reduce his fat. The interval workout says that the workout should be done on various sessions of 15 minutes. This 15 minute session should be very intense and then after the session a person should take some rest. The metabolism process starts in those 15 minutes.

5. Practice Low Impact Exercise

There are a few exercises like running on asphalt floor or skipping. These exercises leave a lot of impact on the muscles of the body specially the feet muscles. These exercises lead to muscle breakage and it tears down the stamina to work out more. It is advisable to do intensive exercise but a low impact one. The exercises of this nature are cycling, swimming and running on elliptical machines.

6. 15 Minutes Interval Workouts

To reduce fat early one should to cling to interval workouts. These are the short and heavy sessions of workouts. In a shorter span of time one can lose more as compared to the regular cardio workouts. If a person does 20-30 minutes of interval workout, 2-3 times in a week then he reduces more as compares to 30-60 minutes of daily cardio workouts. The best part of interval workouts is that one keeps losing the body fat even after the workout session is not in the progress. The fat metabolism process is alleviated and it keeps happening for 48 hours after the work out session.

7. Change The Pattern And Time

Our body gets used to a workout. If a person is doing a particular kind of exercise at one particular time, on each and every single day, then the exercise will stop showing results after sometime. Let us take an example to understand it better. If a person is doing 3 sets of 10 squats each at 8am in morning, on a daily basis then after a month or so the body will get used to the pressure of 10 squats at 8am and thus will stop showing any results. That is why it is advised that a person should keep changing the number of sets he is doing, change the time of exercise and also the kind of exercise, from time to time. The change will give better results.

8.   Body Toning In Interval Exercise

After the 15 minutes exercise session, all the stubborn fat is reduces and the skin is not visible as a loose skin. The interval workouts help in development of muscle in place of fats. This is the reason that, even after burning lot of fat the skin becomes tight as it has been transformed into muscles.

9.   Exercise In Cool Area

It is commonly known and accepted that a person cannot exercise a lot in high degree temperature an. It is advised that the exercise should be done in cooler areas. If at all a person has to work out in high degree then he can cool his temperature around his neck and can work out for more time even in high degree. Wear an ice strap around neck region or wear a wet handkerchief around a neck region and run in treadmill. The duration will definitely increase vis s vis non cooling exercise.

10. Wear Comfortable Clothes

During work out wear something which does not absorb heat from outside and store in the body. for example if someone wear black color clothes during workout then this color cloth will absorb all the radiation from sun and will not reflect back. This will increase the heat within the body. The body is anyways heated up because of heavy workout and then if it socks more heat from outside then it will be dangerous for body. One should always take care of clothes and wear loose and light color clothes.

Conclusion

You now have the tools to workout without worrying about travelling or having access to a gym. You can workout anywhere at anytime. All you need is your bodyweight and determination. With these workouts, you can take your fitness to the next level by learning how to get fit, lean muscle mass and burn fat faster than traditional cardio workouts with minimal time.

You will be amazed at what your body is capable of doing when you challenge yourself with new workouts for fat burning. These workouts will help you burn maximum calories and get lean muscle mass too! If you would like to learn more about the secrets of fat burning then go here my website Bodyweight Cardio Training. You will learn more about fat burning workouts without needing to spend hours on the treadmill or run on a track. You can get fit without having to spend hours a day. You will learn the secrets of bodyweight cardio training to get lean muscle mass and burn fat in minimal time. So why wait. It's time to start your bodyweight cardio challenge now. Goodbye boring workouts for fat burning! Hello bodyweight cardio training for lean muscle mass and fat burning.

CPSIA information can be obtained
at www.ICGtesting.com
Printed in the USA
BVHW011520250321
603178BV00033B/562

9 781802 244304